ORDER
ON THE
COURT

ORDER
ON THE
COURT

Pro Beach Volleyball:
A Rally for Respect and Recognition

Tom Burke

ORDER ON THE COURT

Printed in the United States of America.

FIRST EDITION

LCCN: 2008932327

ISBN-13: 978-0-9817530-9-6

For information, please contact:

Olympic Proportions Press
P.O. Box 300
Burtonsville, MD 20866
www.orderonthecourt.com

To purchase additional copies of this book, visit us at www.orderonthecourt.com

*For all the professional beach volleyball players
who possess the courage and patience to
follow their dreams, pursue their passions,
and fight the good fight each and every day.*

Contents

One

Ladies First

Leaping towards each other, the two beach volleyball players ecstatically embraced. As they collapsed onto the soft sand, they hugged each other ever so tightly – their bikini-clad bodies intertwined. Thousands of courtside spectators and the millions of television viewers cherished this moment – long to be remembered among all Olympic Games celebrations. This beach volleyball final was indeed the *hottest* event of all at the Athens 2004 Summer Olympic Games.

Misty May-Treanor (known as Misty May until her November 2004 wedding) and Kerri Walsh basked in the moment... on top of the world. Their longstanding dreams of winning the beach volleyball gold medal were finally attained. "I remember just looking at Misty after we won and freaking out. It was just this uncontrollable reaction to what just happened," recalled Walsh. "We've taken a lot of flak about it, but I'd do it again in a heartbeat."[1]

It had been a long, arduous journey for these Golden Girls to reach this pinnacle – a goal of all Professional Beach Volleyball players. After finishing fifth at the Sydney 2000 Olympic Games, the determined May-Treanor set her sights on Athens. Seeking a change, she split from her partner, Holly McPeak and invited Walsh for a tryout. After witnessing Kerri's performance as a star player on the fourth-place United States Indoor Volleyball Olympic team in Sydney, May-Treanor saw her beach volleyball potential. From their initial practices, she recognized that she "wouldn't want to choose anyone else as my teammate."[2] Walsh, however, doubted her ability to transition to the much different beach game and second-guessed her decision to accept May-Treanor's offer. "I looked like an idiot at first, I really did," she said, reflecting back to how clumsy she felt on the court, not to mention feeling self-conscious about her 6'3" lanky body in a bikini – a stark contrast to her indoor uniform: jersey and shorts. "I was literally embarrassed to practice in front of other people, and I was kind of intimidated by the beach."[3]

As they launched their partnership in 2001, many women players were eagerly signing up to compete on the revived Association of Volleyball Professionals (AVP) domestic professional tour. May-Treanor and Walsh, however, could not reach agreement with management on sponsor-related contract clauses. So they took their bikinis and balls overseas to compete on the prestigious international circuit led by the Federation Internationale de Volleyball (FIVB) – an organization that conducts the Olympic Games beach volleyball qualifying process. Despite their minimal experience as a team, they amazingly finished within the top ten teams at each of their nine FIVB tournaments. Then, in 2002, they continued their success, winning five of the eleven FIVB events they competed in. Simply phenomenal.

When the 2003 season began, they faced a grueling 13-month Olympics qualifying period that would determine the 24-team field for the Athens Olympics. Walsh and May-Treanor were jet-setting across the ocean to compete in two tours: the FIVB and the AVP, which they returned to after agreeing to relaxed contractual terms. During this time frame, this top-ranked juggernaut swept the competition, winning an astonishing 89 straight matches, a record to this day. They were excited about qualifying for the competition on this world stage once more – this time together. "We had been beating people down for four years. We wanted to show the word what we had and without a doubt, by winning the gold medal," said Walsh.[4]

It almost didn't happen. In June 2004, May-Treanor suffered an abdominal strain, similar to an injury that haunted her in Sydney. While May-Treanor focused on resting and rehabbing, Walsh competed with other players to keep in shape, causing everyone to wonder if their Olympics bid was in jeopardy.

As the Olympics competition began in mid-August, though, a recovered and fit May-Treanor emerged in Athens. The tournament favorites were back, proving to the world their strength and dominance. They swept all their matches leading up to the gold medal finals on that memorable August 24 evening.

The beach volleyball arena was rocking. The 10,000 hyper fans who packed the beachside stadium were marveled by the animated announcer, the pulsing techno-pop music, and the gyrating "Fun Girls" dancers, whose shiny, silver bikinis glistened under the bright lights. Everyone was getting amped because these matches would decide the gold, silver, and bronze medal winners. In the opening bronze medal match, the second USA team of McPeak and Elaine Youngs clawed their way to victory, edging a stubborn Australian team in three games. This emotional win further pumped up an already juiced Walsh and May-Treanor, who seized the court for the gold medal contest to face a nemesis Brazilian team. "The energy was so electric out there. I fed off it so much," said Walsh.[5] In a lopsided two-game sweep, Walsh and May-Treanor prevailed – a culmination of a dominating and undefeated run among the best in the world. "It's like a dream come true," the fist-pumping May-Treanor said as she dusted herself off from the alluring embrace that captivated the world.

Soon afterwards, the trio of top finishers stood atop the colorful, three-tiered podium for the awards ceremony on this warm and beautiful evening. As the two U.S. flags were raised on the stage, the emotional "Star Spangled Banner" reverberated through the stands, generating a gold rush of chills. After the anthem's final note, the four teary-eyed Americans, wearing the champion olive branch wreaths along with their medals, raised their arms in triumph. This wonderful night was indelibly etched in the memories of those fortunate to have witnessed one of the most poignant wins in Olympics history. May-Treanor said that to this day, "I still get goose bumps seeing our flag being raised as we stood on top of podium."[6]

Befitting any Olympics gold medalist in a popular sport, the Golden Goddesses returned home as celebrities. As soon as they landed on U.S. soil, they hurried to the MTV Video Music Awards show in Miami to present the Viewers' Choice award. Then, this overnight sensation hit the talk show circuit, appearing on NBC's Tonight Show. During the next few months, their popularity rocketed and the corporate world took notice. Although not chosen by General Mills to appear on a Wheaties box, each soon signed endorsement contracts with such companies as Gatorade, Nautica, and Speedo.

May-Treanor and Walsh soon received such prestigious awards as the 2004 U.S. Olympic Spirit Award from the United States Olympic Committee and the 2004 Sportswomen of the Year award from the Women's Sports Foundation. The accolades continued...

Sports Illustrated's 2007 Women Athletes of the Year and the Gatorade 2008 League of Clutch, which honored them among such sports greats as Derek Jeter, Peyton Manning, Maria Sharapova, and Abby Wambach. And entering the ranks of pop culture, they were featured on the fitness-oriented cover of *Parade* magazine in January 2007 with NBA star Lebron James.

Though taking time to bask in their new celebrity status, May-Treanor and Walsh firmly set their sights on their next goal: winning another gold medal in the Beijing 2008 Summer Olympic Games. But the road to Beijing has been a bit bumpy. First, as in any partnership, they had their share of ups and downs. In 2006, they spent less time hanging out together off the court and began to drift apart. Walsh explained, "The communication between Misty and I wasn't so great, and there were a lot of little problems that could have split us up." This falling-out led to some heart-to-heart talks near the end of the season. "We found out where we stood. I think it really strengthened our relationship," said May-Treanor.[7] Second, they had to withstand the grueling 14-month qualifying period for the Beijing 2008 Summer Olympics, with domestic and international tour events held week after week. "It's like my head is here and my body has no idea what's going on. It definitely takes its toll, especially the international travel," said May-Treanor.[8] Third, both have been nagged by injuries: May-Treanor's problematic knees, and Walsh's troublesome shoulder that required surgery in November 2007.

Still, May-Treanor and Walsh have continued to dominate the world of Pro Beach Volleyball, becoming the winningest women's team on both the AVP and FIVB tours, where they are the reigning world champions. "Kerri and Misty are the stars people come to see. People from all walks of life come to see the best female team in the sport," said McPeak.[9] Their indisputable fitness, fiery competitiveness, and fun-loving outlook personify everything that is beach volleyball. Their fame has attracted thousands of new fans to the sport each year.

Even before that one magical moment shared by Walsh and May-Treanor in Athens, U.S. Beach Volleyball has always been energized by Olympics success. Ever since beach volleyball's inaugural event at the Atlanta 1996 Olympic Games, Americans have cornered the gold medal market. Karch Kiraly and Kent Steffes stood atop the podium after winning the men's gold in Atlanta, and Dain Blanton and Eric Fonoimoana captured the top prize in 2000 in Sydney. Every four years, fan interest soars due to this Olympics windfall – a spike that other second-tier professional and Olympic sports like tennis and boxing can only dream about.

Beach volleyball, born in the United States, has so much going for it. The sport is vested in strong tradition, hailing from its casual, grassroots California beach heritage. In recent years, this action-packed and fun-filled sport has been tagged as an "Extreme Sport," joining the ranks of edgy, lifestyle sports like snowboarding, mountain biking, and skateboarding whose popularity is surging. Also, beach volleyball's sex appeal stands out among all sports, thanks to beautiful babes in bikinis and buff beefcakes in boardshorts.

And yet, the sport that glittered like a jewel in the Athens night is still barely a speck in the broad landscape of American sports. Despite the Olympic-sparked upsurge in beach volleyball popularity, the AVP's attempts to ride this momentum and take its pro sport to new levels have sputtered. Pro Beach Volleyball's turbulent history in the 1980s and 1990s, when men dominated the game, still haunts the quest to this day. Unable to cast off these remnants of its damaged reputation among sponsors and television broadcasters, the strapped AVP still grapples with financial survival, while fighting to establish any kind of credibility and respect amidst a crowded sports entertainment business.

The disorder and uncertainty within Pro Beach Volleyball rifles through the ranks of the AVP players, many of whom have Olympic aspirations. Scrambling to survive in a sport they love, they fight the good fight. These talented athletes, the equivalent of pros in any major sport, devote considerable time and energy to the game – practically on a year-round basis. Each and every season is an uphill climb for these players, who are not guaranteed a salary by the AVP and receive minimal support from the USA Volleyball organization for overseas competition.

Not even Walsh and May-Treanor are immune to the hurdles, although they certainly can tolerate these headaches more easily from the lofty vantage point they have rightfully earned. As a humble team respectful of its male forefathers, they want the whole sport to succeed as badly as the lowest-ranked players do. They sincerely hope that their achievements and notoriety will open a door to fame and fortune for future players. "A lot of men have helped pave our way. We feel like we're ambassadors for the game. We want to carry the momentum onward," explained May-Treanor.

Walsh and May-Treanor, along with everyone else who love beach volleyball, recognize that the time to move forward is now – or never. As the Beijing 2008 Olympic Games approached, the Golden Goddesses had locked a high seed. This Dream Team was once again favored to win despite competition that has greatly improved since Athens. "It's important that we kick butt in Beijing, so we can push the sport to the next level," said Walsh.[10]

Yet even with another women's gold medal, or a valiant attempt at one, the AVP cannot rely solely on this Olympic boost. The 2008 season is "make or break" for the AVP. A strong start is vital to pro-actively propel itself upwards and onwards in the way Walsh envi-sions. Is the current AVP management ready and willing to tackle this challenge, a truly ambitious effort that may very well require a full-scale makeover? And will Pro Beach Volleyball ever earn a spot on the American sports podium?

Two

A ROLLING WAVE

Pro Beach Volleyball is nowhere to be found on the American mainstream sports radar, and no one close to the sport is happy about it. The big three – football, baseball, and basketball – pull in tens of thousands of fans for every game, with millions watching on television. Other than the Olympics, that kind of attention is a distant dream for this sport. "Pro Beach Volleyball is still seen by a lot of media and sports fans as a niche sport and doesn't receive nearly the attention of the traditional 'stick and ball' sports," said Toby Whitmoyer, a brand director for Jose Cuervo Tequila, one of the AVP's steadier sponsors.[1] During Pro Beach Volleyball weekend tournaments, only a few thousand fans fill the stands whose capacity is not much greater than that of a large-sized high-school stadium, and just several hundred thousand viewers ordinarily catch the limited live-televised broadcasts.

This inability to capture the public eye leaves those closest to the sport scratching their heads. Unlike the major sports, volleyball is a lifestyle activity that attracts people of all ages, and can be played on a variety of surfaces – hardwood, asphalt, grass, or sand – making it very convenient for everyone. Over 46 million Americans play the sport, either indoor or outdoor.[2] Although the beach volleyball spin-off can be conveniently played with teams of three, four, or six players, the most popular format is doubles. Even to the casual observer doubles is easy to understand and exciting to watch – just two players on either side of the net who score points when their opponents fail to keep the ball in play. It's as simple as that. And with bare-chested men and bikini-clad women flying around the court chasing balls, what's not to like?

However, many onlookers simply don't take beach volleyball seriously. Many argue that the festive vibe, also rooted in other extreme sports, detracts from the sport's genuineness. Others consider the non-contact, safe sport to be lame and as a result, boring. Diving into the soft sand while wearing no protective equipment except sunglasses is far removed from the hard-hitting rumbles on Astroturf or hardwood that many find entertaining. For these spectators, beach volleyball deserves to get sand kicked in its face. Last, some feel that images of oiled and tanned, scantily clothed bodies bouncing all over the court is barely proof of a demanding sport. "Maybe it's too sexy for people to legitimize," said Elaine Youngs. "Maybe all people see are bikinis and bare backs and think it's a big barbecue out here. Who knows?"[3]

In defense, those who play beach volleyball or follow it passionately will argue that the sport is demanding, one requiring the 200 pros to keep in shape year round. To those who question this sport, they say, "Let them try walking in the hot, deep sand under a searing sun for an hour, and see how quickly their opinions change." Picture this activity ratcheted up several notches – that's what beach volleyball players face when competing in hour-long matches several times a day during tournament weekends. "Fundamentally, beach volleyball is the same as indoor volleyball. But you throw in the sand, the wind, the sun, and the fact that there's two of you on the court covering the same area, it's pretty intense," said Kerri Walsh.[4]

Indeed, Pro Beach Volleyball in the U.S. has an image problem. Fair enough. But why? To understand the roots of this dilemma, it's helpful to look back at the sport's roller-coaster history.

Beach Volleyball History 101

The traditional six-person indoor sport of volleyball, with 800 million players worldwide, was founded in 1895 at a YMCA in Holyoke, Massachusetts. Laden with elaborate regulations about player positions, substitutions, and refereeing, volleyball is indeed formal and structured. For many, though, the sport is enjoyable and exciting – despite the regimented format.

Beach volleyball, in comparison, is a renegade offshoot. The sport's roots date back to the Roaring Twenties, a decade known for prosperity and hope. In California, beachgoers and vacationing families, who were tired of building sand castles and tossing footballs, adventurously rigged makeshift nets on Santa Monica beaches. And within the shadows of the amusement park on "Pleasure Pier," beach volleyball was born.

Seeking more challenges not offered by the six-person format, energetic (and likely bored!) players left the confines of the enclosed gym behind and formed teams of two instead. Since the 1930s, this doubles style has been adopted as the truest version of the sport. With two players striving to cover the entire court of slippery sand, this "anything goes" format sharply contrasts with the "stay-in-your-spot-and-perform-your-own-role" six-person routine.

Within the next two decades, interest in the sport began to spread worldwide, with beach volleyball informally surfacing on beaches in such countries as France and Bulgaria. While on the home front, the sport became better organized, despite its cult-like status. Venturous players conducted informal tournaments on such California beaches as Santa Monica's Sorrento and Malibu's Will Rogers State Park. Here, men's matches spanned the entire day and often stretched into the evening hours, with car headlights beaming onto the championship match court. As a sidelight, beauty pageants were also held on-site, where women paraded along the beach in corset-like swimsuits in full view of wolf-whistling oglers.

During the 1960s, the Hippie Generation decade, interest in beach volleyball climbed. The counterculture creed "Turn On, Tune In, and Drop Out" was the motto many lived by, as an escape from the rat race and the Vietnam War. The times they were a changing, and beach volleyball fit right in. The sport's followers retreated to the beaches, toting tents and surfboards, to catch the weekend action at such cities as Manhattan Beach, Santa Cruz, and San Diego. After each exciting yet lengthy day, the beach bum players and fans returned to their tents or vans to party through the night listening to the likes of Bob Dylan, The Who, The Beach Boys, and The Beatles, who once even dropped in at Santa Monica to bump the ball around while on their U.S. tour. "In many ways, beach volleyball was a refuge from mainstream life," said Kevin Cleary who began competing in 1978.[5]

Despite the "anti-establishment" sentiment of the times, in 1965 the California Beach Volleyball Association (CBVA) began organizing tournaments and establishing rules, many of which stand to this day. Back then the strategies were simple: hang back on defense and dish up whatever comes at you. From dawn until dusk, top players like Ron Von Hagen, Ron Lang, and Gene Selznick (the first to be credited with spiking the ball on a consistent basis) constantly competed.[6] And the reward for their first-place finishes? The honor of competing on center court or, sometimes, even a case of Pepsi – whose bottles could be returned for some extra pocket change.

The Spirited Years

Acclaimed beach volleyball historian Art Couvillon appropriately labeled the 1970s beach volleyball era as the "Spirited Years."[7] Early on, the freewheeling men competed each year in a dozen or so tournaments that were managed by the frugal CBVA. The athletes worshipped this grassroots sport that was organically evolving as part of an easygoing lifestyle. Wearing bandanas to secure their sun-bleached locks, and brightly colored short shorts (no speedos, thankfully), these bronzed guys lived and loved the game. Back then, these die-hard beach rats, on limited incomes themselves, could not afford a new beach volleyball. They treasured any ball they could find – waterlogged, torn, or misshapen – anything to practice and compete with at events.

The ladies at the beach were looking to play ball too. As a nod to the rising women's liberation movement, the CBVA began including them in its lineup. The women's season schedules were initially shorter, and their weekend events were conducted at separate locations. But as the '70s progressed, more tournaments were held each year. With this upsurge, the women became more confident in their play and in their venturesome swimsuit selection (one-piece evolving to bikini), a reflection of this emboldening era.

As more tournaments were added each season, this billowing wave began surging up and down the California coast and even splashed into Nevada and Hawaii. During this laid-back era, every year the competition improved and the sport's popularity grew. For any weekend tournament, the players would show up on Friday – just in time for the start of Happy Hours. The arriving fans would soon follow them to the bars, after saving prized spots courtside using blankets and lawn chairs as overnight markers. After a night of pre-tournament celebrating (any excuse to imbibe!), "Players slept on beaches because they were too drunk to find a hotel room or could not afford one," said Matt Gage who competed in over 70 events during the 1970s.

Then, bright and early on Saturday, the whole gang stumbled to the courts, where splintered 4' x 4' poles, sagging nets, and ungroomed sand served as a welcome mat for this carefree lifestyle. While the tournament progressed throughout the day, more fans arrived – typically standing shoulder to shoulder, three to four rows deep around the perimeter of each court. The sun-baked partying continued, with buried beer kegs fueling the spectators, as well as to the players who often claimed that downing beers was strictly for medicinal purposes – the prevention of muscle cramps. Whatever! Then, after fighting their way on the first day through several matches (some lasting up to two hours), the players would again drink the night away. After once more crashing on the beach while carefully avoiding high tide, they'd return to the courts, hangovers and all, to compete with an eye to the finals.

During tournament play on Sunday, the competition would intensify despite only the glimmer of a non-monetary prize for the victor. When a losing team was knocked out of the event, they would usually referee the next match – sometimes involving the pair they just lost to. These pissed-off and now beer-chugging refs would occasionally hold grudges. "This would lead to lively arguments before, during, and after the match," recalled Sinjin Smith, a member of the Volleyball Hall of Fame.[8] These events ordinarily ended before nightfall. But when they didn't, the remaining teams would settle the championship by a variation of the "rock, paper, scissors" game. In any case, as Jim Menges, who won 40 tournaments in this decade, recalled, "The winners would receive a free dinner, a volleyball, or a pitcher of beer."

But soon, this carefree vibe was rocked by a commercialism undercurrent. These beachside events began to lure sports promoters and sponsors who saw value in supporting this wild partying sport. They envisioned an emerging, untapped audience to which their products could be marketed. In 1974, the sport turned professional. Winston Cigarettes sponsored a CBVA tournament in San Diego, providing $1,500 in prize money and much-appreciated free samples at a time when cigarettes were still considered "cool" and not so unhealthy. Quickly following this "sin" product lead, Olympia Beer and Jose Cuervo Tequila soon tapped into the spiritedness by also hosting events that were flanked by their oversized, inflatable bottles. The emerging professional beach volleyball bandwagon was gaining momentum... increases in sponsor funding drove greater prize money, which attracted more players, who competed in front of larger crowds.

In 1976, a cunning entertainment promoter, Event Concepts Incorporated (ECI), snagged this growth opportunity and formed a men's Pro Beach Volleyball tour. At its "World Championships of Beach Volleyball" tourney, ECI introduced scoreboards and paid referees to the sport. Held in Santa Monica, this tournament attracted 30,000 fans who witnessed such stars as Von Hagen,

Menges, Gage, Steve Obradovich, and Chris Marlowe compete for a record-setting $5,000 in prize money. Each year thereafter, ECI cranked up the prize money and the number of tournaments. The capitalism gears were soon set in motion with more sponsors lending their names and financial backing to this tour.

The Transformation Years

At the start of the 1980s, the once casual, domestic beach volleyball tour began to evolve into a businesslike machine. The grassroots style started to burn away, and there was no turning back. ECI further expanded the Pro Beach Volleyball tour, venturing outside the confines of the sport's California birthplace into Florida, while upping the overall, seasonal purse into the tens of thousands. More sponsors jumped on board, such as Miller Brewing Company, Jeep, and Coppertone, who were all intrigued by the sport's action, sex appeal, and beach scene. One notable company, the sports equipment corporation Mikasa Sports, was seeking a market for its newly designed volleyball made of synthetic, suede-like material. A sweet financial deal with ECI was soon inked, and this unique ball was adopted as the "tour" ball for use at all events. But this agreement was not met with open arms. The players passionately objected to this harder and heavier ball that replaced the favored leather, Spalding-produced ball that they had competed with for years. Despite these complaints, ECI refused to budge – requiring the pros to play with this artificial albatross.[9]

With more money on the line, the men competed even more intensely. The matches began to last longer, occasionally up to four hours – a marathon by today's one-hour standards. As a result, tournaments stretched well into the evening hours, with some never finishing. These time-consuming events cost ECI more money to conduct, and the TV networks balked because these protracted matches would often overrun the allotted broadcast time slot. Accordingly, ECI switched from a "sideout" to a "rally" scoring format. Due to this change, a point was earned with each new play regardless of which team served the ball. Matches then could be completed in an hour or so, cutting the average playing time in half. But the players, stubborn purists at heart, myopically objected to this quick-paced format that replaced the long-lasting, "play-until-you drop" style, thereby setting the stage for a showdown.

As beach volleyball transformed into a business benefiting from sponsorships, the men, who used to play just for the fun of it, began to land corporate deals too. These money-hungry guys were not only fighting on the court for prize money, but off the court by competing for sponsors such as Renault, Honda, and Jose Cuervo Tequila for endorsement contracts (that were nominal when compared to athletes' deals in other major sports). Yet these professionals soaked up all this newfound fame and played the game – in more ways than one. Many adopted an outrageous, fun-loving style, as an offset to their businesslike demeanor. They quickly became celebrities on and off the court during this footloose decade. Rolling into a beach town for a tournament, they eagerly awaited a rowdy weekend of competition and celebrating, as a carry-over from the 1970s.

The undisputed showman Tim Hovland personified this enthusiasm to the hilt. Bolstered from six-figure deals with sponsors like Renault who gifted him a set of wheels, he brought this confidence onto the court where his unbridled arrogance endeared him to all – except his fiercest competitors.[10] This 6'4" volleyball god partied with fans during tournament nights and relied on just enough sleep to carry him through the weekend event. During this decade, his commanding presence and loudmouth taunting of opponents swept him into dozens of championships – to the amazement of many. His persona was a perfect match for a game that was becoming more physical – with players spiking more often, and penetrating the net to block attacks (due to a newly introduced rule). Powerful plays and jabbing gibes – that's how they rolled back then. "If you got in my way, you were going down," said Hovland, smack-talking to both pissed-off opponents and entertained hecklers.

As the sport's popularity surged, the strict Federation Internationale de Volleyball (FIVB), the world's formal governing body for indoor volleyball, began to take notice. These suits traveled from their Europe headquarters to the California beaches to witness the men compete at the events held by the newly-formed Association of Volleyball Professionals (AVP), while also inspecting the women at tournaments run by the Women's Professional Volleyball Association (WPVA). Upon their return, they decided that this sister sport should be also regulated and organized at the international level. By 1987, the FIVB loosened its necktie and began conducting its own beach tournaments – choosing Rio de Janeiro, Brazil for its opening event.

The Golden Years?

Pro Beach Volleyball was the bomb as the 1990s began. Tens of thousands of fans were drawn to these weekend carnivals at beach towns in California, Florida, and New Jersey to see both men and women professionals play. For example, the California vacation town of Santa Cruz welcomed everyone each season. With its picturesque cliffs bordering the courts, suitably wide beaches, and diversionary amusement pier, this beach volleyball magnet was the ideal backdrop for weekend partying, swimsuit contests, and of course, the competition. Packed like sardines, fans surrounded the courts awaiting the high-fiving players who had to squeeze through the packed crowd to reach their match on time.

Soon beach volleyball began to catch on worldwide. While recognizing the sport's attractiveness and commercial appeal, the FIVB organization recommended to the stodgy International Olympic Committee (IOC) that the sport be included in the Summer Olympics. And on September 21, 1993, the IOC added beach volleyball to the Atlanta 1996 Olympic Games schedule. This decision to debut the sport in its birth land surprised everyone and was especially welcomed by the U.S. athletes who were among the best players in the world. Looking back, Karch Kiraly, a two-time gold medal Olympic indoor volleyball player, said, "It's something I never dreamed would happen. I never thought beach volleyball would be a part of the Olympic program. But all of a sudden it was."[11]

Just three years later, the whole world watched this inaugural Olympic sport on television. This eye-popping event, featuring athleticism, fun, and sex, injected energy into the Olympic line-up and drew high ratings. Well-conditioned players from dozens of countries wore the officially designated uniforms of bikinis as well as jerseys and swim trunks. The main stadium, erected in a suburban park, hosted several thousand zealous international fans. Brazilian trumpeters, Australian drummers, and American flag-wavers cheered their countrymen to the medals round. Although the U.S. women's teams narrowly missed winning a medal, their fellow men's teams ruled the competition on their way to the finals. There, Kiraly and Kent Steffes swept Mike Dodd and Mike Whitmarsh for the gold medal in this monumental event (that led to the eventual addition of other extreme sports like snowboarding and BMX cycling to the Olympic Games program). Afterwards, the International Olympic Committee (IOC) acknowledged it had a winner on its hands – as evident by the large crowds, the rousing competition, and the multitude of puritan complaints lodged about the prurient attire. While reveling in this afterglow, the IOC began to prepare for an even better show at the upcoming Sydney 2000 Olympics, with the pledged backing of eager media and sponsor corporations.

In the U.S., Pro Beach Volleyball reached its all-time peak in 1996. While primarily relying on funding from its sponsors, the player-run AVP myopically increased annual prize money to record-setting levels. Many of these enterprising men wore two hats – a beach volleyballer who showed up to compete and rake in tens of thousands of dollars, and a profiteer who quickly flipped this prize money into real estate deals or stock market investments. With certain tournament wins paying out $100,000 (the equivalent of 25,000 cases of soda), they soon became millionaires. Unfortunately, this greed proved to be financially disastrous in the latter 1990s for both the AVP and the now-defunct WPVA.

The Rebuildng Years

As the new millennium opened, the American pro sport was surprisingly struggling. Puzzled fans, noticing the demise, were comforted by the United States' stellar performance at the Sydney 2000 Summer Olympic Games. There four teams finished within the top eight, qualifying under a new tournament system fully controlled by the FIVB.

On the heels of this success, interest in the domestic pro sport began to rekindle in 2001. A former AVP executive, Leonard Armato, returned to lead the sport, by then on the verge of collapse. During his initial reigning years, the Pro Beach Volleyball tour conservatively and gradually got back on its feet – offering prize money far below levels in the previous decade while gradually attracting sponsors and television networks. And by combining both men's and women's competitions, the AVP lured fans to return to the sport to cheer on those athletes who stuck with the tour during its downfall, as well as newcomers like Misty May-Treanor and Kerri Walsh.

Then, of course, their gold medal victory in Athens spiked another post-Olympic fever. More star college graduates switched from their victorious indoor teams to form beach partnerships in hopes of achieving similar prominence and fame. For example, former Pepperdine University standouts Brad Keenan, Sean Rooney, and John Mayer transitioned to the AVP after graduation and immediately challenged the top, elite teams.

Players like these adopted a workmanlike approach to the pro game, focusing on financial survival while using their time efficiently. "Back in the old days, the pro players would often play 300 days a year on the beaches. Now it's more of a job with two to three hours of drills at the beach in the morning, then time in the gym in the afternoon," said Hovland. By hiring coaches, trainers, and nutritionists, as well as agents, these athletes were serious about succeeding in an unsteady pro sport that is, for many, a full-time job on a part-time pay scale set by the tight-fisted AVP.

Because more people are taking up the sport, beach volleyball courts are now popping up everywhere, like the gophers in the "Whack-A-Mole" carnival game. And not just around the U.S. but in such far-off places as Croatia, Egypt, and India. As a result, the omnipotent FIVB has accepted beach volleyball registrations from over a hundred countries whose teams compete in its tournaments. By further stretching its tentacles beyond its base in Europe, the FIVB is now holding tournaments in the Far East and in the South Pacific – not only for the elite who seek Olympic Games berths in its "Main Draw" tournaments, but also for those less experienced who compete in the "Challenger" and "Satellite" breeding ground events.

And so it is that this little sport, born on the beaches of California, has stretched across the entire world. But what kind of international respect is granted to this birthplace? Not much, in recent years. Although the FIVB has recently conducted events in Canada and Mexico, this tour is not likely to make a stop in the U.S. any time soon. Due to longstanding tensions between the AVP and the FIVB involving the Olympic qualification process, scheduling conflicts between their tours, and AVP's ambition to expand overseas into FIVB territory, the poorly attended 2003 FIVB event in California may very well have been the last.

Three

JUSTICE IS NOT SERVED

"In this sport, the Americans are just another country now, not the country," said Sinjin Smith.[1]

Both indoor volleyball and beach volleyball have thrived on American soil well before the rest of the world took notice. The time-honored traditions, the longstanding history, the well-ingrained pride – all should be enough to both sustain a strong domestic foundation, and promote excellence on the world stage. However, in recent decades other countries have leapfrogged over the U.S. This American foothold has surprisingly eroded, overtaken by powerhouse teams from Brazil, China, and Russia as shown by results in the sports' pinnacle, the Summer Olympic Games. Case in point, the U.S. Olympic Men's and Women's Indoor Volleyball teams have not won an Olympic medal since 1992, and the American medal count for beach volleyball has been surpassed by Brazil. What gives?

In the way of background, the International Olympic Committee (IOC) requires that each country establish a National Olympic

Committee. In America, it's the United States Olympic Committee (USOC) whose proud mission is to "Support the U.S. Olympic and Paralympic athletes in achieving sustained competitive excellence and preserve the Olympic ideals."[2] Each Olympic Games sport in the U.S. is governed by a National Governing Body (NGB) that is funded, in part, by the USOC. For both indoor volleyball and beach volleyball, USA Volleyball (USAV) "works towards provision of ample opportunity, quality opportunity, and equality of access for every resident of this diverse nation."[3] The organization consists of over 210,000 active members ranging in age from 8 to 80, with the vast majority competing indoors. Given this weighted membership base and its deep-rooted philosophy, the USAV has unceasingly backed and advanced the indoor game at the expense of the beach game. The majority of members on the bureaucratic USAV's Executive Committee and Board of Directors have traditionally hailed from the indoor sport – laden with its extensive protocol, bylaws, and regulations.

Chief among the USAV's goals is "To win gold medals in every international competition."[4] To this end, the USAV has traditionally supported the U.S. National Indoor Team in its Olympic quest, ever since the sport was first contested at the Tokyo 1964 Olympic Games. Male and female players practice, work out, and receive medical treatment and counseling at the prestigious U.S. Olympic Training Center in Colorado Springs, Colorado. Then, during breaks from their training, they retreat back to their comfortable dorms for meals, rest, and relaxation. They need not worry about their room and board expenses, nor any overseas travel costs at Federation Internationale de Volleyball (FIVB) tournaments. Based in part on funding from the USOC, the USAV covers these expenses and even pays salaries to the players, indicated Nicole Davis, member or U.S. Indoor National Team.

Has all this physical, psychological, and financial backing paid off in terms of Olympic indoor volleyball glory? Not so much. Since the Tokyo Olympics, eleven Summer Olympics competitions have been held. And the result? The U.S. men's and women's indoor teams have only earned five medals, with the last podium finish at the Barcelona 1992 Olympic Games. This disappointing medal performance has continued far too long, and impatience by the USOC and the national volleyball community is at an all-time high.

Flip now to the beach game – considered by many of these USAV "old-schoolers" to be a rebellious outlaw and a second-class spin-off. "Beach volleyball is seen as the bastard stepchild by the USAV," according to an experienced insider wishing to remain anonymous. The legitimacy of this sport, with half-naked players bounding around, has always been questioned by the old-fashioned USAV. Not even has Olympic Games success been able to change their stance. Since beach volleyball's debut in the Atlanta 1996 Summer Olympics, the Association of Volleyball Professionals (AVP) men's and women's pairs have also won five medals, tying the overall U.S. indoor total in just three Olympic Games competitions. And with its gold medals in each of the three Olympic Games, beach volleyball has single-handedly helped the USAV meet its ambitious gold medal goal.

This unexpected gold mine was, of course, warmly welcomed by the USAV, which graciously accepted all praise despite devoting little effort to beach volleyball. Realizing it had a winner on its hands, it slowly began to elevate the sport by fostering a juniors program to develop young athletes during the 2000s decade. Camps, clinics, and tournaments have been conducted to "provide grassroots programming as well as identify top beach volleyball athletes for 'high performance' development programs."[5]

Unequal Justice

That's all well and good, but the Olympic-caliber, Pro Beach Volleyball athletes have continually been "dissed" by the USAV, whose support has been deplorable. Is an Olympic Training Center available for beach use? No. Do these star athletes receive room and board compensation? No. Are coaches provided to these athletes at no charge? No. Three strikes and you're out, USAV!

Deplorable conditions have continually shackled beach volleyball Olympic hopefuls. First, they have always been responsible for their living expenses, such as food, lodging, and transportation. Second, they have paid for all training, and coaching costs. Third, when competing overseas to qualify for the Olympics, they have traditionally covered their own airfare and lodging expenses, in hopes of receiving some compensation from the Federation Internationale de Volleyball (FIVB) or the USAV. Then, once on-site at a FIVB event, each player has served as a medical trainer for her teammate's ailments and as a coach by videotaping competitor matches for study during breaks. With all these demands, not borne by other competitors whose countries provide complete support, it's truly amazing how these disadvantaged players have continued to compete so well internationally.

However, the USAV's passing of the buck had to stop sometime, and the AVP and its players united to drive change. On numerous occasions assistance from the USAV was sought. For example, in April 2003 a working committee was formed so that both organizations could regularly meet to better promote beach volleyball in the United States. Rebecca Howard, then Chief Executive Officer (CEO) of the USAV, sheepishly announced, "We feel lucky that the AVP has offered a connection to their already established program. It's not news that the USAV has not been very successful in promoting this well-loved discipline of our sport."[6] What an understatement! But despite the best intentions, this partnership fizzled.

Next, in March 2005 an agreement was signed between the USAV and the AVP to jointly form a "Beach Volleyball Council," to focus on "formulating plans and implementing programs with respect to the growth and development of beach volleyball in the United States." This planned cooperation sounded promising, with goals of "creating a National Beach Volleyball Team" (similar to the indoor model) and "assisting USA beach athletes in winning Olympic Medals."[7] But, the subsequent CEO Doug Beal guardedly said, "Any initiative that is going to be undertaken by the Beach Volleyball Council that has any Olympic or funding implication (relative to USOC support) is going to have significant USOC involvement and will have to be implemented within USOC guidelines and with USOC approval."[8] Needless to say, because of this callous stance, this partnership was also temporary. To this day, few current USAV board members even recall this ill-fated attempt.

Although these failures have been rationalized by each organization in a politically posturing way (aka "formal finger-pointing"), many professional AVP players believed that the USAV had let their sport down. Clearly, the top beach pairs, who were well known on the FIVB circuit, were not getting domestic respect. But what bothered these players the most was that the beach game stood the best chance to land medals. Even Karch Kiraly, a member of the 1984 and 1988 U.S. Olympic gold medal indoor teams, referred to the USAV's historical underpinning of beach volleyball as "somewhere between total apathy and lack of respect."[9]

AVP v. USAV

Disgusted with the lopsided USAV support that has favored the indoor game over the beach game, the upset players and the sympathetic AVP decided to jointly pursue legal action. Meeting in late 2005, they discussed their options and came out locked and loaded. In January 2006, in an exceptionally rare move within Olympic circles, official papers were served. An Article VIII legal complaint was filed by the AVP and 28 of its players – including Misty May-Treanor, Kerri Walsh, and Kiraly. In this 40-page filing requiring a USOC response, the complaint alleged that the USAV was negligent by: offering no meaningful financial aid, providing minimal scouting and coaching help, and denying beach volleyball sufficient representation on the USAV Board of Directors. The complaint further boldly demanded that the USAV be stripped of its role as the NGB for beach volleyball.

In short, Pro Beach Volleyball was calling out the USAV big time for its neglect and inaction. The lawyer for these complainants, John P. Collins, quickly put a calculated spin on this action. "We tried to resolve this without filing a complaint. The status quo of 100 percent indoor and zero beach is not acceptable. The beach sport needs the attention to maintain its dominance and position in the world. We're prepared to do what it takes to make it happen," he said.[10]

A shocked USOC, already rocked by the Salt Lake City 2002 Olympic bribery and corruption scandals, was forced to take action. At first, this formal organization responded with public relations representative Darryl Seibel tersely stating, "I don't know if you will see a quick resolution to this. We have procedures to deal with these complaints."[11] The stubborn USAV also began to legally position itself. Beal initially replied, "We filed to dismiss the complaint on several grounds. The vast majority of the issues raised in the complaint are without merit." Through this (in)action, the USAV would not have to reply to every allegation made in the filing – a time-consuming and reputation-threatening ordeal. Collins soon countered, "The beach sport needs the attention to maintain its dominance and position in the world. We're prepared to do what it takes to make it happen."[12]

Despite the defensive stance, the USOC requested the USAV to address the cited complaints in the legal action as part of its cleanup and restructuring process – dictated to most all NGBs in the wake of the Salt Lake City 2002 Olympics scandals. To propel these USAV changes, the USOC added the leverage of withholding the funding of hundreds of thousand of dollars from the USAV if it failed to adhere.

While heeding the legal complaint's assertions and the USOC's directives, the USAV finally began to budge. Ali Wood, a retired women's Pro Beach Volleyball player, was hired in February 2006 as a new Director for the International and High Performance Beach Program. She was tasked with "coordinating programs that directly support the athletes who are trying to qualify for the Olympic Games." As she launched her role, Wood said, "I think I have a good relationship with most, if not all, of the players and I understand that what the top players need might not be what an up-and-coming player needs."[13] To her credit, several beach players joined the USAV Executive Committee and Board ranks, such as elite-level AVP player Tyra Turner who was elected as an International Beach Player Representative. She stated that more help has been fortunately provided to the pro players in 2007, "such as monthly travel stipends, health insurance, on-site medical care, and scouting of competitors at international events." To ensure these players took advantage of these new offerings, Turner was the first to remind them, "I fill the void by informing players about the benefits they are entitled to. Many don't even know."

Cleaning House

Seeing the writing on the wall, the guilty USAV Board of Directors, at its annual meeting in January 2007, made a monumental decision to restructure itself by cutting its voting membership in half and mandating a fairer representation of indoor, outdoor, juniors, and grassroots representatives. Rose Snyder, the chair of the committee tasked with selecting applicants for this new Board, said, "It is our goal to put together the best team – a team that will lead and govern the organizations and... put personal allegiances and agendas aside for the greater good and long-term interests of the sport."[14] You Go Girl! Looking back, Angela Rock, a Board player-representative and former AVP pro said, "The meeting was scary and thrilling. We made history. This was the best thing to happen to the USAV in a really long time." This leaner and representative Board, complete with two beach representatives, is to be formed soon after the Beijing 2008 Olympic Games.

The USAV also decided to change its outdated bylaws to streamline its processes and reduce bureaucracy, thereby, it is hoped, freeing up more dollars to fund beach volleyball. However, most importantly, the USAV is finally challenging itself to champion not only a greater awareness about beach volleyball but to begin treating both sports *somewhat* equally. "Our primary goal is to grow volleyball at all levels all across the country," said Beal. "We have dedicated funding and resources to showcase beach volleyball, especially at the grassroots level."[15] Towards that goal, the USAV has established the U.S. Open of Beach Volleyball. With assistance from the recently retired Kiraly, USAV held the championships in September 2007 at Huntington Beach, California where a few hundred players competed in 15 divisions. Looking ahead, Kiraly said, "Our hope is that we will be able to bring this great game to more people with a nationwide grassroots approach."[16]

The Article VIII filing has since been dropped, and the AVP and players have rested their case. But the jury is still out about the USAV's future support for Pro Beach Volleyball players. The steadfast Beal still downplays the turbulent period when the USAV's future was in jeopardy, while slowly resigning himself to the imminent reorganization. "It's not a situation where we screwed up and need to make significant changes. But the changes we're making have the likelihood of being positive for the sport."[17] These couched words from the helm are not overly encouraging for Pro Beach Volleyball.

Let there be no confusion. The USAV faces challenges in elevating beach volleyball to the level befitting its strong heritage. Besides the USOC squeeze, the FIVB is strongly encouraging each country's NGB to create a "national beach volleyball circuit and integrate programs for Beach Volleyball players like the (indoor) Volleyball players."[18] With pressure from both the USOC and the FIVB mounting, the USAV must stand behind beach volleyball at all levels – from the youth learning the game to the pros pursuing Olympic glory. The AVP and its players can only hope that these steppingstone improvements will steer even greater assistance. Misty May-Treanor is both optimistic and realistic, "The USAV has come aboard and things have changed since I first started," she said. "It's like anything else. It's a learning process for them, after promoting the indoor sport for so long."

However, without this backing from the U.S. Olympic hierarchy, U.S. professional beach volleyball clearly is in jeopardy, if reliant on the shaky track record of the AVP.

Four

FROM 100K PAYOUTS TO IOUs

Guarding the entrance to the Beach Volleyball 1984 World Championships, the striking players brandished picket signs: "Where's the Money" and "F--- Event Concepts," as strands of the union fight song, "Solidarity Forever," blasted from a boom box:[1]

> *"They have taken untold millions that they never toiled to earn,*
> *But without our brain and muscle not a single wheel can turn.*
> *We can break their haughty power; gain our freedom when we learn*
> *That the Union makes us strong."*[2]

Over this three-day weekend event, such high-profile players as Tim Hovland, Mike Dodd, Sinjin Smith, and Karch Kiraly protested the Event Concepts Incorporated (ECI) promoter's petty prize money payouts and control over the future of beach volleyball. As lower-ranked players crossed the picket line to compete, these scabs were confronted with insults and spit. Even the arriving fans felt this angst, greeted by reminders like "The best players in the world are not participating in the tournament today."[3] Despite the warning, close to 30,000 ventured inside to see these second-rate teams struggle at this Redondo Beach, California site. Other fans hung out in solidarity with the boycotting players – some of whom passed the time drinking, and flipping the bird to passersby. As a result of this mutiny, the quality of competition was pathetic – almost laughable – and ECI's stranglehold on the sport began to loosen.

Birth of a Player Nation

The promoter's unilateral switching to a rally scoring format and mandating the use of a synthetic ball had fueled much of the anger. Enraged players, clinging to tradition, objected to being dragged down this commercialism path. Kevin Cleary, a well-respected player on the tour, met with ECI management in May 1983 to discuss player concerns. But ECI refused to budge.

Carrying this stubborn posture back to the players, he began to seek support from those wanting more say in the sport's future. A meeting was soon held among the players and a sports agent, Leonard Armato, to discuss their options. Due to this growing frustration, these participants voted unanimously to create a players' collective. On July 21, 1983, the Association of Volleyball Professionals (AVP) was formed. According to Cleary, the elected President, several guiding principles formed this charter:[4]

> ➤ Preserve the integrity of the game

> ➤ Participate in the running of tournaments (e.g., scoring system, equipment)

> ➤ Allow more opportunities for individual sponsorships

> ➤ Issue greater prize money

Looking back at this monumental period, Armato said, "The athletes had no professional assistance and had no rights whatsoever in connection with the evolution of the sport. There was little money in it."[5] Almost 20 years later, those words would have a different ring to Armato, but in this pivotal moment of the sport they perfectly reflected his sentiment.

With these ambitious intentions, the AVP's newly formed Board of Directors tried to partner with the ECI staff in 1984. But the powerful ECI ignored this upstart unit's advances. That infuriated the players even more. So, the headstrong AVP conducted its own tournament in July 1984 at Malibu, California during a break in the ECI schedule. The ECI firm winced at this slap in the face.

The event was a success, fueling greater AVP mojo that led to the World Championships strike just two months later. While grasping these small victories, the AVP quickly became recognized as the ambassadors for this professional sport. Using this momentum, the inspired group negotiated a partnership agreement in October with Group Dynamics, a promoter of pro tennis tournaments eager to expand its business by managing the tour. Fearlessly taking a step further, the AVP won another battle by convincing ECI's top tour sponsors, Miller Brewing Company and Jose Cuervo Tequila, to instead sign up with Group Dynamics for the upcoming season.[6] The fuming ECI staff saw its position start to erode and soon bit the dust – never to return to the pro beach game again. As expected, the AVP quickly nailed this coffin shut by resurrecting the favored sideout scoring for the 1985 tournaments. At this early stage, the foundation for the emerging, player-run AVP was being cast. This bold insurrection, coupled with shortsighted passion, would unfortunately plant a seed for eventual turmoil.

By 1987, the increasingly confident AVP deliberated about taking over the tour from Group Dynamics, as proposed by Armato, the Executive Director who led the organization while reporting to the Board. The AVP reasoned that, by managing the events itself and dealing with sponsors directly, expenses would be cut, and sponsor income could be freed up for greater tournament purses. The top sponsor, Miller Brewing Company, recognized the AVP's contributions to the sport, and favored the AVP running the entire tour. To that end, Miller Brewing Company severed its partnership with Group Dynamics. In December, a three-year contract between Miller Brewing Company and the AVP was signed, granting the AVP 100 percent ownership rights to the tour, and revenue from licensing, merchandising, and television.[7] As a further vote of confidence, Miller Brewing Company agreed in 1988 to foot $4.5 million in prize money, and cover all the AVP's expenses – an astonishing agreement, even by today's standards!

Buffeted by Miller Brewing Company's support, Pro Beach Volleyball surged during this decade:

> ➤ Average per-tournament prize money rocketed from a mere $7,000 in 1980 to $65,000 in 1989

> ➤ Annual tournaments increased from seven to twenty-three

> ➤ Fan attendance per event soared from the thousands to the tens of thousands

> ➤ Yearly incomes of top players sailed well into the six-figures – compliments of prize money and sponsor endorsement income

In sum, the men's AVP tour quickly matured into the latter 1980s with an eye fixated on revenue and the various means to attain it. The previously footloose and casual events in the 1970s yielded to regulated, corporate-influenced tournaments. Stadium seating supplanted beach chairs, paid referees substituted for assigned players, and beer sponsors "illegalized" buried beer kegs. Soon, additional sponsors such as General Motors and Coppertone jumped on board this income-driven train. These endorsements boosted both prize and sponsorship income for the players, assuring that two of the AVP money-grubbing "guiding principles" would be met.

During this growth period for the men, the women's professional sport was starting to settle. The Women's Professional Volleyball Association (WPVA) began holding tournaments in 1986. Many top players like Linda Chisholm and Nina Matthies competed in these events, earning about 10 percent of what the men raked in.

Changing of the Guards

Having survived the transitional 1980s, the AVP was feeling fat and happy as the 1990s rolled in. However, right from the outset, turmoil within the management ranks erupted. The AVP's Board of Directors and Armato parted ways for reasons that, to this day, are still controversial and closely guarded by insiders. Some assert that Armato was ousted due to a disagreement over accounting practices; others state that he resigned due to a disagreement over his compensation package.

In any case, Jeff Dankworth was hired in 1990 to fill the Executive Director opening. Known for his strong marketing and sports management talents, Dankworth quickly began catering to the media and sponsors. During his five-year reign, he initially negotiated a contract with NBC to broadcast events live, and then reached agreement with Miller Brewing Company to renew its contract for another four years. "Miller bought a lot of advertising time on

NBC and this allowed AVP tournaments to get a great deal of air time. It bankrolled the tour for several years," recalled Mike Dodd. In the wake of this deal, a feeding frenzy ensued. Nissan, Old Spice, Nestea, and Evian all quickly signed up to also sponsor this exciting sport.

Given this new direction, the pro sport was getting hotter, with more than two dozen outdoor tournaments held each year along the coasts of California and Florida, as well as in such inland cities as Milwaukee and Cincinnati. And, in an unusual move at the time, Dankworth organized a mini-tournament in New York City's Madison Square Garden in February 1993. Over 200 tons of sand were delivered for a single-day event watched by 12,000 excited fans.

During his tenure, tournament attendance, television coverage, and sponsorship income rose. While relying on these revenue sources, the AVP awarded $4 million in prize money in 1994. For certain events the winning team earned $100,000, approximately four times the first-place payouts of today. Several old-school beach players such as Kiraly, Smith, Dodd, Kent Steffes, and Randy Stoklos suddenly became millionaires. They enjoyed these short-term riches and limelight while ignoring how this prize money was obtained. "We were in heaven back then," recalled Dodd.

But move over, beach boys. The large payouts attracted even more players to the sport, with many shifting from collegiate, indoor glory to pro beach stardom. Due to this influx of educated players, schooled in the formalities, structure, and regimen of indoor volleyball, the "come as you are," carefree beach volleyball lifestyle further eroded. Through disciplined practices and systematic training, these players budgeted their time and reaped benefits come tournament time. This "take the money and run" businesslike manner, in which many merely put in their time without giving back to the sport, would eventually work against them and the sport they loved.

Hot and Bothered

In contrast, while the men's tour was gaining momentum, the financially struggling WPVA was barely surviving, bouncing paychecks and losing its television contract with ESPN.[8] Sensing their frustration and while eyeing market growth, Dankworth lured several women away to compete in AVP events alongside the men. Stars like Holly McPeak, Angela Rock, and Nancy Reno left the WPVA to play on the 1993 AVP tour. This exodus splintered an already unstable WPVA, which was upset by this solicitation of many of its top players. However, these recruited ladies soon regretted their decision. Their contests, in effect, became sideshows – subordinate to the men in stature and in prize money. In 1994, the women were frustrated that the AVP paid out prize money that was only half of what the WPVA was awarding, and far less than the men's purse. Barbara Fontana, who remained loyal to the WPVA, said, "Back then, the climate was not good. The AVP promoted these matches as exhibitions and the pay was unequal." But, this AVP tactic only lasted two seasons, with the recruited women returning to the WPVA.

However, just as this nexus of sport, entertainment, and marketing worlds was successfully converging, Dankworth abruptly resigned from the AVP due to family commitments.[9] In 1995, the AVP then hired Jerry Solomon, head of a sports and entertainment firm, as the next Executive Director. Due to his minimal background with beach volleyball, many observers considered this hiring to be an ill-fated step. He was considered by many to be a hack, a wannabe who just didn't fit in. However, what he did bring to the table, besides his cronies that he hired, was a notable professional tennis management background. This overconfident outsider tried to manage Pro Beach Volleyball similarly to how the pretentious Association of Tennis Professionals tour was administered. Banking on this experience, he made two income-generating moves that were revolutionary for the beach game in this era, yet common in tennis as well as other sports. First, admission was regularly charged at outdoor tournaments, a change that quickly alienated fans. Second, control was relinquished by the AVP via franchising out its tournaments to local promoters.

These moves infuriated the AVP player leadership, who were admittedly not schooled in the business side of sports. The player-run Board of Directors lacked marketing savvy, not knowing the difference between a volleyball spike and a ratings spike. Therefore, the players succumbed to this "blind leading the blind "scenario, as the AVP continued losing money. Infighting erupted between Solomon's management team and the Board about what direction the sport should take. "It seemed like Solomon never had the players' complete trust. But to be fair, as the sport grew, there were more and more players who wanted to take rather than give," reflected then Player/President Dan Vrebalovich.[10] Million-dollar sponsor payments were quickly flipped to greedily stoke the tournament prize money treasure chest. This selfishness, buffeted by strong egos, enraged the corporate sponsors who felt their money was not being properly channeled into advertising the tour and their products.

Despite these growing concerns, the sponsors were distracted in 1996 as all eyes focused on the Atlanta Summer Olympic Games, with its inaugural beach volleyball event. At this peak, the AVP awarded itself a record-setting $4.5 million in prize money for a 23-city tour where the traveling party was unleashed at each stop. Soon after the Olympic Games, close to thousands of fans turned out for the Manhattan Beach tournament where, in a packed stadium, everyone welcomed and congratulated the two victorious U.S. teams returning to the tour.

However, while the egotistical AVP was basking on its pedestal, its debts were accumulating. Although this organization's financial records were not made public, many insiders realized that the tour was bleeding a red tide of financial losses for several years. One sign: any income that remained after prize money was issued would need to be earmarked to cover expenses. Needless to say, bills went unpaid. For instance, the Integrated Sports International (ISI) firm, which sold lucrative AVP sponsorship deals to Sunkist, Swatch, and BMW, was owed a six-figure debt. At the time, a frustrated ISI representative Frank Vuono said, "The sport is healthy, all the rest of it is what's screwed up."[11]

By 1997, the runaway Pro Beach Volleyball sport could not be reined in. Even as the tour began to self-destruct, it was still selfishly paying itself over $3 million in prize money, while its debt quickly burgeoned to this same level. The now wary AVP began plunging from its mountaintop – careening down a treacherous financial path, and dodging lawsuits from franchisees and liens from suppliers along the way. Enough was enough. The disgruntled Miller Brewing Company stopped buying advertising time on NBC. Because this funding was yanked, NBC pulled the plug on its own coverage by the season's end. According to NBC Sports Vice-President Jon Miller, "They never grew as a business organization. It was always run by the players for the players' benefit, and not putting money back into the organization really hurt them in the long run."[12]

Solomon's three-year stint ended later in 1997 with a "mutually agreed-upon resignation" or, as some have dubbed, a firing. The frustrated Solomon, acknowledging the calamitous conditions, said, "Players just can't be management and labor at the same time. That's an impossible task in any sport."[13] The AVP, ignoring its condition, was unknowingly sinking deeper into a financial abyss.

Baptism Under Fire

Enter Harry Usher, former U.S. Football League commissioner, hired for the 1998 season by the somber AVP Board to lay down the law. As Executive Director, his primary challenges were to keep the AVP financially afloat by reducing prize money, to seek an investment partner, and to restructure the multi-million dollar debt. "It was pretty chaotic when I came in, but I think the players are facing up to what has to be done," Usher observed. "It has been kind of a hard dose of reality for some."[14]

In 1998, in the aftermath of Miller Brewing Company's tapping out, there was a big-time exodus of disillusioned sponsors who, with just cause, pulled out with their money bags in tow. In their wake, Usher recast the debt and paid off creditors who swallowed a tough pill by accepting payments well under what they were owed. Furthermore, the tour was forced to slash costs, with the overall prize money for the season dropping to $1.3 million, down from its $4.5 million peak just two years earlier.

But not all players were willing to go along for this ride. Steffes, nicknamed by many as the "poster child for greed," smacked the AVP with a "derivative" lawsuit. Through a legal action of this type, the complainant seeks "compensations for a loss that the party has experienced due to gross negligence or mismanagement."

Although details about this specific lawsuit were not publicized, the multi-millionaire Steffes was apparently unwilling to take a pay cut. Furthermore, he did not hesitate to call out the AVP, its players, and its business partners. Through public statements, he frequently trash-talked the AVP for its "misconduct" – namely, the lowering of prize money. These continual smackdowns annoyed the AVP, and in April, Usher warned this notorious bad boy to "cease and desist" because he had violated contract provisions that restrained players from disparaging the organization.[15]

Unlike the past, when players were practically guaranteed thousands of dollars for just stepping onto the court, these shocked athletes were now competing for IOUs… issued from themselves. The now austere tour had lost its charm, and puzzled fans began to wonder what had happened. Soon word got out about this downturn, and fans remained home. And stay away they did, with only a thousand attending the San Diego tournament.

In one of his last acts in his short-term gig, Usher regretfully put the AVP up for sale. "The AVP is a name that's worth something. It's a monopoly on the best players in an Olympic sport," he declared.[16] The offered deal? One million dollars and payment of all outstanding debts. Surprise, surprise – no takers! "Everyone knows this isn't a hard property to market," said the departing Usher. "It just hasn't been run particularly well."[17]

Later in 1998, sports marketing firm owner Bill Berger (a former Marketing Director of the AVP from 1988 to 1990) and Dan Vrebalovich (a former AVP President) jointly approached the struggling AVP with a plan for reorganization and repair. The two were immediately designated as the Chief Executive Officer and the Chief Operations Officer, respectively. Would this pair be the first "sports marketers," among the many who failed, to save the tour? By now, the players were apprehensive, uncertain about where the AVP was headed and about their futures. Their previous ally, Vrebalovich, was now cracking the whip on them, trying to turn the AVP around during this precarious period.

Laying down the law from the start, the new AVP brass slapped a three-year suspension on Steffes in November 1998 for his continual bad-mouthing. "It was bad timing to be making remarks as the AVP was trying to turn itself around. There's been more than enough infighting over the last several years and it's important that we get back to having fun and running a business, which is the sport of Pro Beach Volleyball," explained Berger.[18]

They next studied the financial books that bulged with close to $3 million of debt, and realized the AVP had become a victim of its self-serving excesses. At wit's end, they helplessly decided to throw in the towel – filing for a Chapter 11 bankruptcy. In turn, the AVP was granted relief from its debts and permitted to forge ahead with a planned financial reorganization. A deal was then struck with the players who agreed to forgive several hundred thousand dollars in unpaid prize money, and with the creditors who consented to receive compensation less than what they were owed.

Touch-and-Go

While this court-ordered reconstruction was underway, the future of the AVP still looked bleak. As a last resort, the restructuring AVP began negotiating with an investment firm in early 1999. Berger and Vrebalovich, as minority investors, partnered with a surprisingly interested venture capital firm, Spencer Trask Securities, to purchase the AVP out of bankruptcy – its only chance for survival. And for the first time since 1983, the players were not running the organization.

During the next 1999 and 2000 outdoor seasons, the AVP scaled back, organizing only a dozen men's tournaments and limiting prize money to a mere $1 million. As a sign of the times, the players were promised "per-diem" payments – a set prize money payout regardless of how they finished. Women were invited to six of the 1999 events, and they jumped at this chance to compete after the WPVA's own collapse in 1998.

While barely managing to stay afloat during the years surrounding the millennium, the AVP could not effectively market nor organize its tournaments. Unlike the bustling tournament scene in the mid-1990s, the tour had now deteriorated into a seedy carnival on its last desperate day. The tournament grounds were skeletal, with the customary dazzling AVP banners, inviting sponsor tents, and bustling television crews of the glory days now history. Everyone – fans, players, sponsors, and broadcasters – worried if this now struggling tour would survive.

Although these executives were still optimistic, the major investor, Spencer Trask Securities, was still nervous – dreadfully so. They shuttered the AVP headquarters in California and warily assumed control from their formal New York City offices.[19] With the AVP's 2001 season on the horizon, the profit-minded firm was way outside of its comfort zone. Since the purchase, the tour took on more debt each year. Tired of hanging on, more sponsors departed, choosing the contract non-renewal or termination route. Due to the drought of sponsor income and the burgeoning debt, the bankrupt AVP was near collapse. Skeptical fans were understandably slow to return to these events. Similarly, players like Olympic gold medalists Dain Blanton and Eric Fonoimoana, as well as such promising stars as Dax Holdren and Stein Metzger, decided to play in the upstart Beach Volleyball Association – a new competitor of the AVP.[20]

Pro Beach Volleyball's downturn during the last decade of the 20th century was certainly unexpected. Based on the feuds between management and the players, many questioned whether this "Association" with its inherent partnership and coordination undertones was still a fitting label for this organization. Most insiders and onlookers agreed that the sport required a rebirth. "There's been too many people that have come into this sport looking for quick money and just sucked it dry," said Vrebalovich. "What we need is someone who wants to get down and dirty and build it."[21]

Five

LIFEGUARD TO THE RESCUE?

While surveying the tantalizing scene at the Sydney 2000 Summer Olympic Games beach volleyball venue, Leonard Armato was amazed at the sport's immense popularity. The stadium, bursting with thousands of cheering, dancing, and singing fans at the picturesque Australian Bondi Beach, was rocking in time to the pulsating music. During these breaks in the fast-paced competition, he couldn't help but wonder why this sport was dying on its home front. Looking back, the determined Armato said, "I have to resurrect this thing. It's not right that it's popular around the world and there's nothing in the place it started."[1] Soon afterwards, he began contemplating a return to his sports management roots.

During the AVP's rise and fall in the 1990s, Armato was managing the star-studded careers of such top athletes as Shaquille O'Neal, Kareem Abdul Jabbar, and Oscar de la Hoya. As their agent, he savored the lucrative dealmaking, big-time sports excitement, and Hollywood lifestyle. Yet, he still kept his feet wet in the professional beach volleyball scene – assisting the Women's Professional Volleyball Association (WPVA) with its marketing plans while dating one of its star players, Holly McPeak. While witnessing the AVP's near-death experience and the WPVA's extinction, he was well aware of all the controversy and demise rifling through the sport. Would he want to leave this glamorous world to retreat to a barren landscape bereft of excitement, money, and fame? And could he save this flailing AVP organization?

In early 2001, just months after the Olympic Games, the AVP was gasping for life and needed a savior, pronto. Armato returned to his AVP roots, just in time. His company, Digital Media Campus, was awash in earnings from sports agent income. The millionaire negotiated a deal on May 31, 2001 with the welcoming investment firm to buy out the AVP. At the time, Spencer Trask Securities senior manager Spencer Segura said, "I don't think there's ever been a better shot than this. If this doesn't work, I don't know who will ever want to try it."[2] With the start of the season only days away, the two parties agreed that Digital Media Campus would acquire 80 percent of the AVP in a low multi-million dollar deal. "I felt there was this huge opportunity to reinvigorate the sport in the U.S. and reestablish the AVP as the dominant force in beach volleyball," said Armato.[3]

So, like a scene straight from the *"Baywatch"* TV show, this lifeguard ran in to save the sport. But what could be done? To find the answers, he had to look backwards.

Not on My Boat

First on deck were the players – the heart of the tour. While relying on his volleyball rapport and marketing savvy, he outlined controversial conditions to steady the ship. Right off the bat, Armato threw a life preserver out to the women – among them his fiancée, McPeak. In recent years, the frustrated women were floundering in rough waters, seeking to compete on whatever tour they could. The WPVA tour had already gone down, and the newcomer Beach Volleyball Association was taking in water. Therefore, by inviting them on board, Armato rescued the women and tried to stabilize the sinking AVP ship.

During the previous decade, of course, the AVP had tried this merger, but the women hated the second-class treatment. This time around, however, Armato leveled the playing field, guaranteeing them equal prize money and events, beginning with the 2002 season. Through this combination, he reasoned that the sport could reap greater media attention, the fans could better follow the tour, and sponsor investments could be optimized. But enough with the corporate mumbo-jumbo smokescreen. By including these bikini babes on the scene, the sport's sex appeal would be heightened.

In another provocative move, Armato sought to end the player defiance and excesses of the past by requiring each athlete to sign a contract. Among the strict stipulations: displaying sportsmanship, treating sponsors with respect, acknowledging AVP ownership of licensing rights to the players' images for marketing, and not competing on other tours.

Armato also instituted the use of the new international beach volleyball rules to ensure consistency between the domestic and international games. The Federation Internationale de Volleyball (FIVB) in 2001 implemented rally scoring, reduced the court size, and allowed let (or net) serves for its international events and for the upcoming Athens 2004 Olympic Games. Given these introduced rules, the game would be speeded up and become more fan-friendly. Rally scoring could cut the match competition time in half. With the court size reduced by approximately 20 percent, players could cover their side more easily, thereby keeping the ball in play and elevating the action.[4] And "legalizing" let serves would also ensure a continuation (rather than a stoppage) of play.

What did the men, who were well accustomed to earning millions and who favored the old style of play, think of all these changes? After all, it was their boat that was being rocked and weighed down with more passengers. Many were completely caught off-guard by these quickly introduced changes that required flexibility, patience, and understanding. "It was definitely a little helter-skelter," said the soft-spoken Dain Blanton.[5] For other players, these intrusions were a total buzz kill. Beach volleyball purists, such as Karch Kiraly, wanted to retain the prolonged, sideout "play until the sun goes down" game that represented strength and endurance. For him, this climate was a déjà vu – for he was among those who revolted in 1984 against the ECI promoter's rally scoring format. Others, like AVP millionaires Kent Steffes and Adam Johnson, bolted for the door. Adjusting to both the sizeable pay cuts and the new rules was just too much for these veterans.

Despite these objections, the resolute Armato stood his ground. Amazingly, over 100 men and women players signed up, including young newcomers who grew up with the evolution of "extreme sports" and favored a faster pace with more exciting play. As a whole, the players recognized these changes were required for the sport to succeed. Even the apprehensive Kiraly had a change of heart. "Leonard laid out a strategy for us, and the players are on board. We want to bring the AVP back to its glory years," he proclaimed.[6] And the feeling was mutual. Looking back, Armato said, "We were delighted that the players embraced their role as our partners in rebuilding the AVP."[7]

Patching Things Up

With the athletes aboard, Armato charted his visions for controlled growth and survival within a business plan that outlined financial and operational goals, and the methods to achieve them. He then focused on rebuilding the wrecked corporate ship, which had recently leaked much-needed revenue as sponsor and television companies fled. When reconnecting with these corporations, Armato had a twofold purpose: to restore their blemished image of the AVP, and to implore them to rejoin the tour. While relying on his keen marketing prowess, he fit the bill as the best herald. "You need a guy with vision and unbridled optimism. Leonard has that," said Rick Welts (former NBA Properties President).[8] Through back and forth negotiations, the cunning Armato coaxed a few sponsors to sign up for short-term deals, and NBC to begin broadcasting a handful of events. "Now, with a three-year plan, the right players and sponsors, we've put it on life support and have tried to give it a life of its own," boasted Armato.[9]

The transitional 2001 season allowed Armato to breathe some life back into the drowning AVP. Yet, despite this "kiss of life," over $1 million in losses were recorded that year. To buoy this weak vessel, he corralled financial backing from a group of investors that included Oracle Corporation Chief Executive Larry Ellison, music producer Quincy Jones, and chief executive of Playboy Enterprises, Inc., Christie Hefner. This $6 million dollar investment was used to stabilize the tour and pay off debts still owed to creditors from the previous decade.[10]

Barely afloat in shallow waters, the AVP conservatively stayed the course during the 2002 season by scheduling only seven tournaments that paid out $1 million in total prize money. It further cautiously conducted 10 events (offering $1.3 million prize money) in 2003, and 12 events ($1.7 million prize money) in 2004. While hugging the coastlines, the AVP held the majority of these tournaments within the safe havens of California and Florida beaches where large fan turnouts could be assured and expenses could be minimized. Such inland cities as Milwaukee, Dallas, and Boulder, Colorado – popular event spots in the mid-1990s – were just too risky now.

During this period, the AVP understandably experienced highs and lows, successes and failures – wavy turbulence, of sorts. Everyone was not on the same optimistic page as the AVP, which often wandered from its scripted business plan as well. Revenues from sponsor contracts, tournament attendance, and product sales were trickling in – despite relying on the Athens Olympics as a promotional tool. As a result, when the three-year plan period drew to a close in 2004, the struggling AVP was still losing money. The $12 million reported revenue gained from sponsorships and events was substantially offset by the $9 million in tournament operating costs and the $6 million in selling and administrative expenses. Despite this $3 million year-end loss, the undaunted Armato said, "I am fully committed and focused on running the AVP long-term and building this sport into an extremely valuable sports property that provides an opportunity for many athletes to make a career playing on the AVP tour."[11] This vision would play out differently in just a few years.

In the off-season, a new business plan was devised as a guide for the next few years. Andrew Reif, Chief Financial Officer, explained, "We expect to see improvement in our business if we successfully execute our strategy … to increase our sponsorship base, media platform, and the number of AVP events."[12] Typical marketing puffery, sweet talk for the masses. To achieve these lofty goals, the

AVP would need to attract even greater financial backing to sustain itself, while fueling expansion and profitability objectives.

Pulling Some Financial Strings

Seizing the windfall of interest from the AVP women's medal wins in Athens, a new AVP emerged on February 28, 2005. As part of a complex inter-organizational merger (aka "corporate shell game"), the AVP went public and netted $4.2 million through its stock offering. In exchange, the shareholders who invested hoped to reap such customary benefits as stock value gains and the right to vote on important corporate matters – the latter, a risk that the AVP was willing to take. Thus, the AVP had to be further accountable to all through public filings with the Securities and Exchange Commission. By reporting its operational, financial, and managerial inner workings, certain activities like unique bartering deals, frequent stock awards to officers, and executive comings and goings were no longer hidden from public view.

This influx of capital was soon tapped to seek new markets, attract more sponsors, increase tour prize money, and cover various expenses. For instance, within the new four-year (2005-2008) player contract, the approximate 200 athletes were guaranteed $3 million in prize money, which would increase each year by $500,000, as the events increased by two. Also, new board members and executives, who were hired to steer this new organization, came at a cost – well into the millions in the form of salaries and stock issuances to these newcomers.

As the 2005 season progressed, the players competed in 14 tournaments while confined by the restrictive and unforgiving contract. The AVP was riding a post-Olympic wave of interest and needed to connect with a greater fan base. It soon began bringing its show to inland locations such as Tempe, Arizona and Cincinnati, Ohio where sand was trucked in to form the courts. "We wanted to have a national presence that advertisers could use as a marketing platform," Armato noted.[13]

While the tour was gaining momentum, the AVP stock price failed to take off. In fact, it was drowning. Management, well out of its (financial) league, did not know what to do at first. The stock suffered on the "over-the-counter board" – a lowly, ridiculed system where many small and unknown company stocks are thinly traded, and share prices are more easily manipulated. Its stock, valued at a phenomenally low 17 cents per share, deteriorated into a "penny stock" – complete with all its worthless connotations. To bolster its image and to attract new investors, the desperate AVP pulled some unusual financial strings to boost its value. In December 2005, the company issued a "reverse 10:1 stock split" to boost the stock price by tenfold, to a whopping $1.70.[14] It also established a new ticker symbol, AVPI, to further distinguish its stock, and to cover up this stigmatizing action. Both of these under the radar actions, although legit, were performed to mask its stock market woes.

This operationally eventful year ended in financial disaster, this time with net losses of $9 million. The $24 million in expenses far exceeded the $15 million revenue gained from receiving sponsor payments, selling TV rights to overseas broadcasters, offering "hospitality packages" for corporate VIP attendees, and entering into licensing agreements for AVP merchandise. As a result, the millions gained from the sale of stock were all but wiped out in less than a year's time. And with only $1 million of cash available for 2006, what could the AVP do?

The solution? What else – issue more shares! Sure enough, through back-to-back stock issuances in May and June of 2006, the AVP sold over $5.5 million in stock shares and warrants. This influx of cash was greatly needed to manage its now 14-event tour that awarded $3.5 million in prize money. Hopeful shareholders warily invested in the AVP, despite its limited management track record, high executive turnover, adverse financial standing, and the risky, short-duration sponsor contracts. Caveat Emptor! Through this accumulated capital, the AVP cash balance jumped by several million – much needed for the 2006 season.

Fortunately, as the 16-tournament campaign unfolded, the somewhat financially stabilized AVP further benefited from two revenue sources: sponsors and local promoters. Its continual efforts to attract sponsors began paying off when the upstart "ugly shoe" company, Crocs, signed a multi-year, multi-million dollar contract to be the flagship sponsor. The AVP also resurrected a revenue-generating technique that was tried by its predecessors just before bankruptcy was declared. In this scenario, the AVP "earned" extra revenue money by subletting the managing of tournaments to local promoters for a fee – in effect, selling off parts of its operations. Total 2006 revenue reached a record $21 million, compliments of sponsor payments equaling $17 million. Despite this gain, and management's best efforts, the AVP just missed breaking even, re-porting a financial loss of a "mere" $300,000.

So, there were high hopes for the 2007 season. Given the pre-Olympics year, the tide seemed to be turning for the AVP, with its plans for 18 events awarding $4 million in prize money. Sponsor income, television ratings, and fan attendance had steadily risen. Everyone was hoping for a profitable year – especially the investors who were expecting the stock's value to rise.

But the Board of Directors had different aspirations. Led by Board chairman Armato, they stunningly voted to enter into "An Agreement and Plan of Merger" where Shamrock Holdings, an investment firm owned by the Disney Corporation, would buy out the AVP. These executives were, in effect, returning the AVP to a privately held company status – steering it away from the watchful eye of investors. In support, the suspiciously retrenching AVP stated on April 5, 2007, "This transaction with Shamrock allows us to streamline our business operation and focus AVP's precious resources on building the business rather than public company compliance and raising capital."[15]

Industry-wide best practices dictate that the Board of Directors must exercise control and management over the company and, in theory, for the benefit of the stockholders who are entrusted to this governing group. Yet, the AVP Board decided that each stockholder would have the right to receive, as compensation for this buyout, only $1.23 per share – well below the previous day's close of $1.50, and below the average 2007 stock price of $1.30 per share. Was Big Brother looking out for Little Man? Hell no! This unusual buyout deal, an anomaly in the world of acquisitions, shocked these now seething shareholders – including investment houses, players, and fans – all of whom were getting the shaft, plain and simple.

Mutiny Over The Bounty

So why would the AVP, on the verge of a profitable 2007, sell out? And why at such a discounted price? A very unusual deal indeed. But before the AVP could proceed with this dubious and, some believe, devious plan, the shareholders would need to approve this action. It didn't take long for the outside investors, who fortunately held a majority stake in the company, to countermove with motions to dismiss. The two largest corporate stockholders zipped off memos to the AVP as official complaints. The raging anger beneath these formally worded and filed positions could be plainly seen. The money management firm, Diker Management LLC, which was responsible to its own investors, immediately challenged this decision. "Management has little incentive to seek the highest price for the existing equity as its stake in the company will roll into the new company. This offer is grossly inadequate and the process by which this deal was evaluated is flawed by clear conflicts of interest."[16] An official understatement of what those at the seething Diker Management really felt inside.

Later, in July, the largest stockholder, AmTrust Capital Management, formally charged that, "The buyout consideration does not adequately reflect the value of the company and its growth prospects" and "Mr. Armato's interest ... created an obvious conflict of interest between public shareholders and the buyout group."[17] And the players, many of whom felt they were being thrown under the bus, were also enraged. Todd Rogers, well respected among fellow players as their advocate, stated that the stock options previously issued to the players "will be worthless if this thing goes through."[18]

In response to these challenges and filings, the resolute AVP management, which lacked a strong financial background, was unusually quiet – an extremely passive way to conduct damage control, and a sharp contrast from self-serving accolades it never hesitated to project. This buyout agreement, as part of a secretive strategic plan, was now on the table, complete with its dirty linen for all to see. The AVP was being called out for its underhandedness and stealth, and they knew it. Busted! Despite this uproar, the AVP made even more waves. It had the audacity to send a letter in August to its stockholders inviting them to vote on a proposal to adopt the Agreement and Plan of Merger at a specially-scheduled, late September meeting. Who were they trying to kid?

The stockholders were both angered and amused by this latest stunt. The previously unsuspecting AVP was now anticipating a mutinous revolt, with the majority of stockholders expected to vote against this planned merger. Finally, hoisting the white flag in surrender in early September, the AVP announced, "AVP and Shamrock realized that a substantial number of AVP stockholders would not vote their shares to approve this transaction. Because of this strong opposition, (we) are terminating the agreement." Amato then personalized the action. "While we are disappointed… we are very optimistic about the future of the AVP and the tremendous opportunities available to enhance AVP shareholder value," he said.[19] His earlier pledge about being "fully committed to running the AVP long-term" was now recognized as hot air, and his trustworthiness level had bottomed out among the sponsors, the networks, the local promoters, the players, and the fans. All in all, this ill-fated ploy cost the AVP over $1.4 million, another telltale drain on its eroding cash balance and a hit to its crumbling bottom line.

With this backdrop of conflict, the 2007 tournament season proceeded as best it could. The AVP stretched into even more landlocked cities to attract more fans. However, the preoccupied AVP, with a permanent staff of just thirty employees, barely outlasted another year, overcoming hurdles such as unusual bouts of bad weather that disrupted events and withstanding the disorder brewing within its management ranks.

A New and Bolder Captain?

In the aftermath of the tempest that rocked its boat, the AVP once again reported an annual financial loss – to the tune of $4 million for 2007. Yet, the ever-optimistic Armato looked ahead to a prosperous 2008 season that would be brightened by its own 25th anniversary celebration and, of course, the Beijing Summer Olympic Games. Grasping this momentum, the AVP conducted a large-scale indoor tour – Hot Winter Nights, a series of one-night stands. As a throwback to the indoor arena events in the mid-1990s, a series of 19 mini-tournaments was held in January and February in northern cities that were unaccustomed to the pro beach game but had a strong indoor volleyball following. "This is a chance for us to create more national awareness and exposure and reach more people and grow more fans," said Armato.[20]

Each event, a small-scale version of the outdoor competition, was held in an indoor arena. There, the bottled beach arrived: 200 tons of sand trucked in to form the main court. Each night, four men and four women players competed in a round-robin exhibition leading up to the finals. The AVP utilized the features of indoor arenas well, taking advantage of spotlights, overhead TV screens, and the comfortable seating. Although each exhibition averaged only a few thousand fans, this new tour may be just what the AVP needs to further build its fan base.

"Our success depends on fan interest, so our business could fail, if we are unable to maintain interest in our sport," according to the AVP in its 2007 Annual Report. Just another reminder that this is one ship that will always be sailing through rough and treacherous waters.

Six

IF YOU GOT IT, FLAUNT IT

At past Summer Olympic Games, thousands of fans and millions of TV viewers joined the beach volleyball party each night to gaze at the world's sexiest sport. The audience was certainly captivated, having one eye trained on the competition and the other focused on the underlying sexcapade. Although the skillfulness of bronzed, chiseled men in precariously hip-hugging board shorts bounding and pounding was indeed riveting, it was the sexy women who stole the show. The female athletes, required to wear provocatively skimpy "two-piece uniforms" that are limited in size by Olympic regulations, were ever so closely watched as they jumped and dived for balls.

This multifaceted "exposure" of beach volleyball has taken the world by sandstorm. Beach volleyball trumps all other sports with its sexual vibe. It's all sun, fun, and buns. No other athletes show as much skin. Not the underwater swimmers, not the costumed figure skaters, not the singlet-wearing sprinters. With a wink and a grin, the formerly stuffy International Olympic Committee invigorated these Games, pumping sexual energy into a tried-and-true lineup that included badminton, skeet shooting, and equestrian dressage.

Bronzed physiques with strong arms, taut abs, tight butts, are the eye candy that draw even outsiders to the sport. With all these hardbodies flying around the court – what's not to like? Furtive stares at these players conjure up moments of imagination among athletic-admiring or physique-adoring fans. Many are infatuated by the half-nakedness alone, and the competition, well... not so much. Sex appeal, as anyone can plainly see, plays right into the AVP image.

The men, as the forefathers of beach volleyball, personified the sport in the 20th century. And the former sports agent Leonard Armato, well accustomed to marketing male athletes, created intriguing images that the public could not only identify with, but even idolize. For instance, under Armato's wing, Shaquille O'Neal's popularity soared, both on and off the court.

But despite this track record of male dominance, he challenged his instincts and hooked up the men with the women for the 2001 season. By including women's matches alongside the men's, and while paying out the same prize money, he not only leveled the playing field but also created a wider foundation for growth and interest in the sport.

Handing Over the Car Keys

Due, in part, to the success of the two women's medaling teams in the Athens Olympics, the popularity tide shifted from the ripped and strong males, to the fit and curvaceous females. They soon began to outstrip the men in popularity, landing stares for their athleticism and allure. This attention then spurred more females to compete in the AVP, which, in turn, has improved their overall caliber of play. The men have accepted their backseat position. "The majority of men I talk to appreciate the women and are not threatened by them," said McPeak, who married Armato in November 2001.[1]

So make no mistake – the women are now on top, and enjoying the ride. The women play the game differently than the men. They rely less on strength and power, and are seldom seen drilling jump serves or smashing down potent spikes – two exciting skills that the men bring to the table. Instead, the females use a craftier style of play, relying on deft ball placement and tenacious defense. This finesse contributes to longer rallies that better capture the fan's attention. This long-lasting style is a fresh contrast from the "wham-bam-thank-you-ma'am" men's action whose plays sometimes end prematurely, before the action heats up. In sum, the boardshort-attired men "go big or go home," while the bikini-clad women "tease to please."

The bikini is the most functional and convenient uniform they could compete in, when compared to biker shorts and tank tops, for example. To be sure, each woman has a different comfort level when it comes to revealing her body. As a result, most order custom-fitted bikinis to ensure a satisfying fit, while looking for high-quality fabric, firm bust support, and flexible elastic around the leg openings. "Once you get used to it, bikinis are very comfortable to play in. It does take some research to find the best style and fit," said Nancy Mason, a veteran AVP player.[2]

Do they feel this exposure is gratuitous? Nope. The women are unconditionally steadfast about wearing this bikini as required by the AVP contract.[3] They are proud of both their physical talents and beauty. Thus, apologies for looking sexy are not required. If jaws drop, so be it. As Kerri Walsh put it, "Being an athlete and a woman, you work hard, you look great, you're fit, you're proud of yourself. If you can walk that fine line of not being objectified, that's great."[4]

A She Said, She Said Argument

Despite this blanket acceptance, these females walk a fine line because these obvious sexual overtones prove to be a double-edged sword. On the one hand, at a broader level, images of partially-clothed women athletes are prevalent in the sports entertainment world, and generally accepted by fans as commonplace. For instance, the U.S. World Cup Soccer Team player, Brandi Chastain, is well known for whipping off her jersey and exposing her functional sports bra to an intrigued audience in 1999. And tennis star Serena William's leather-look bodysuit has continually fascinated fans.

On the other hand, staunch feminists and religious fanatics have profusely complained about what they perceive as a blatant selling of bodies. They contend that these disrespectful players are not serving as good role models. That competing half-naked and sexualizing the female body is not at all liberating. That these women athletes are perpetuating inequality. Equal rights extremists even proclaim that "what's fair is fair," and that men should compete in Speedos that also leave little to the imagination. Yikes!

Today's female pro beach players are not the least bit concerned with these dated arguments. They don't feel like they've cheapened themselves by showing off their bodies. They believe that both femininity and athleticism can be packaged for personal and professional success. After all, why shouldn't they be allowed to compete on the court while showing-off their bodies that have been toned by years of fitness and conditioning? If you've got it, proudly flaunt it, many believe, and rightly so. After all, McPeak had her breasts

Playmates, Not Teammates

Overall, the AVP women unashamedly recognize the sport's sexual windfall and graciously accept its impact on the sport. However, the women's ranks have become divisive at a certain level off the court. In 2005, three AVP upstarts surprised the Pro Beach Volleyball world by posing nude for Playboy. Taking this gamble were Amber Willey (advertised as a "buxom brunette with a killer body"), Jennifer Maastricht ("sexy curves fill out this sleek frame"), and Nicole Midwin ("a curvaceous jock rolling around in the sand"). Of course, women athletes posing nude in magazines is nothing new. However, the pictorial spread prompted some players to object to this selling out. "I'm not cool with Playboy. I wouldn't be proud of that. I think bodies are beautiful, but there's a way to show them," said AVP player Rachel Wacholder, a former model.[10] And what was the outcome of this exposure? Since the publication of these photos, only one featured player has continued to compete on the tour, earning only $175 in 2007.

enlarged (much to the dismay of her feminist partner) just in time for her 1996 Olympic Games competition that was viewed by millions worldwide.

But what do Pro Beach Volleyball fans, as a whole, think? A recent, informal Internet survey asked, "How should the dispute over bikini-clad women at beach volleyball matches be resolved?" The results:

➤ What's the problem?   50%   (Liberal-minded respondents)

➤ Lose the Bikinis!   46%   (Men, of course)

➤ Just Close Your Eyes!   2%   (Level-headed thinkers)

➤ Cover them up!   2%   (Prudes)

These players attract male and female fans. First, women can appreciate the hard work and drive needed to achieve goals. Any athletic-minded woman can certainly relate to these athletes who take pride in their bodies — appreciating the effort required to maintain a fit, sculpted body. They realize that being sexy is more about being confident and content with yourself. Therefore, these players serve as great role models.

Of course, men are unanimously attracted to the women players, quite content to stare at and fantasize about these hardbodies. For them, there is no hung jury. Sexy images of tanned and oiled beach ballers romping around in bikinis are not only entertaining, but arousing. The sport does seem to draw its share of male photography buffs who seem to be more interested in the photographic angles of bodies than the strategic angles of play! Despite this overwhelming fascination, there is one disappointment – the absence of wardrobe malfunctions. Such mishaps as an errant top slipping off or a bottom riding up too far are rare because the women are especially careful. "It's going to go places where you don't necessarily want it to go, and you wish it wouldn't, but you get used to it," Walsh noted. "It's a fact of life."[5]

The AVP's Position on Sex

Whatever side is taken, most agree that sex appeal is an indelible part of beach volleyball. It's simply part of the sport's titillating equation. And for the male-dominant AVP that mandates bikinis, its strongly-supported "less is best" approach reels in more fans. On the tour, the AVP claims there is no outright sexploitation. Bruce Binkow, former AVP Chief Marketing Officer, said, "If the commissioner of the LPGA put golfers in bikinis, eyebrows might be raised. But this is not done in an exploitive or premeditated way. We have an advantage because it's organic to the sport, but it's sexy at the same time."[6] And with a wink and a grin, Armato unabashedly said, "Who doesn't want to watch women in bikinis diving around for balls? But the truth is, if you watch them, they're great athletes... wearing bikinis. What's better than that?"[7]

However, the AVP tiptoes a tightrope with this stance. Apart from alienating women who may disagree with this display, the AVP must worry, believe it or not, about losing respect from a male audience too. Because women are now the centerpiece, certain guys may feel that the game is too feminine. They may not want to be caught dead watching what they believe is a lame sport. Even the liberated Gabby Reece, a former AVP player and model, acknowledged that "If girls can play it, anyone can play it. And if anyone can play it, it must not be a real sport for real athletes."[8]

Not surprisingly, as the AVP continues to search for new ways to better market itself, it recently trialed new strategies of "selling" its women players. Why not squeeze this sexual bonanza, a fringe benefit other sports can only dream about, for all it's worth, right? But several well-intentioned marketing tactics seeking to capitalize on these sexy images were the equivalent of trial balloons – busting soon after being introduced.

As one example, the AVP sought candidates for its advertising on billboards and signs that reveal larger-than-life action shots of women diving for balls. Answering this call one time was Logan Tom, a star U.S. Olympic indoor player who appeared on the cover of *FHM* magazine. When Tom switched to the beach game in 2006, the AVP recognized it had a hot commodity on its hands, and soon touted her as its 2007 poster girl. Tom's lunging image was promoted at tournaments via oversized, in-your-face banners –

coincidentally replacing those that showed off her partner, McPeak. But as her summer hype began to build, frustration between the two began to mount and they split up, reportedly over McPeak's frustration with this newcomer's playing style. Tom soon returned to the U.S. National Indoor Team to seek a spot on the 2008 Olympic squad. And her banners? Presumably residing alongside McPeak's, deep inside a dusty AVP warehouse!

Similarly, the AVP's hyping of Team Gorgeous – the nickname for the dreamy team of Suzanne Stonebarger and Michelle More – has progressed haltingly. At tournaments, this pair attracts a large fan entourage for reasons beyond their competitive skills. The AVP should certainly be able capitalize on this sure bet. However, there's been a small problem. These winsome players have been losing more often than not, seldom finishing among the top ten teams. As a result, many are quick to compare them unfavorably to Anna Kournikova, the tennis star known more for her looks than her skills.

The AVP's most notorious marketing gimmick was its issuance of the Women of the AVP Pro Beach Volleyball Tour 2006 calendar. For sure, calendars with near-naked women are consistently hot sellers anywhere. These ladies, posing in even less than what they wear on the court, were caught covering their exposed bodies with whatever was available. The blond Jennifer Boss draped volleyball netting over her torso, the toned Mason clutched a large palm tree leaf across her chest, and the nymph-like Rachel Wacholder covered herself with mounds of strategically placed sand. Although hesitant at first, these 13 semi-nude pros were cool with these sexually suggestive poses. The bubbly Walsh, who was splayed across the cover, later proclaimed, "AVP players are sexy. There's no way around it."[9] Although the success of the calendar sales is unknown, the AVP said "Ta Ta" to any ideas about a second edition (or even a men's version). So, it's likely the remaining calendars now rest in the same warehouse.

No other sport flashes the flesh like beach volleyball. Yet no matter how hard the male-dominant management has tried to capitalize on the sport's inherent sex appeal, their ambitious attempts have ended in pullouts. With this asset lying right in its lap, the AVP should have no trouble marketing this sport. Sex sells. Everyone knows it. But the AVP has yet to turn a profit. Why no commercial success?

Seven

DESPERATELY SEEKING FANS

"All we need is an opportunity to be discovered," said Leonard Armato.[1]

Sports entertainment is a crowded field. On any given day, all over the country various pro sports are holding dozens of games, matches, showdowns, smackdowns, whatever. The fans who follow these sports come in all shapes and sizes, from intense junkies to the occasional onlookers.

The big boys – football, basketball, and baseball – attract the most attention. Compared to these sports, Pro Beach Volleyball is a relative newcomer to the sports entertainment landscape. With its recognition and popularity still low (outside of its core followers), the AVP has desperately competed for a fickle audience that can easily turn its back on any sport at the spur of the moment. To its credit, though, the AVP has identified its fan base.[2]

➤ Upscale, Active, Health-Conscious Young Adults

➤ Trend Setters, Influencers

➤ Under Age 30: 45%

➤ Under Age 40: 70%

➤ Attend/Attended College: 84%

➤ Average Household Income: $78,000

Despite these common characteristics, Pro Beach Volleyball's current followers have different motives for their interest, and as Armato noted, "You have to connect with the fan at every level."[3] A sizeable percentage of its enthusiasts, to be sure, are solely attracted to the sport's sexiness. But, the AVP can only play the sex card so much. Another large segment enjoys the beach party atmosphere, reminiscent of a laid-back, fun-filled summer vacation. However, with so many events being held inland – at parking lots and in tennis centers – the AVP tour has begun to lose this lifestyle luster. Lastly are the volleyball purists, many of whom have played the sport. These hard-core fans enjoy the competition and avidly follow the teams throughout the season. And, believe it or not, these devotees have their eyes on the ball, and not the bods. Therefore, the AVP cannot afford to alienate these loyalists with sexploitation.

But this fan base is far from solid or even definite. Therefore, every chance it gets, the AVP must seek greater recognition by selling itself to the prospective, "casual" fan – a term coined by industry marketers for those who are undecided about a sport. Every sport chases these prized, "undeclared" fans. And getting these candidates to follow beach volleyball is job one for the AVP.

The AVP well realizes its position in the sports world. Team sports, car racing, and golf rule the land, and their spots are untouchable for all the rest that are groveling for greater fame. Pro Beach Volleyball is precariously nestled alongside such sports as tennis and boxing, in the second tier of this hierarchy. Whereas less popular sports like indoor lacrosse, pro rodeo, and bass fishing bring up the rear.

To climb up this sports hierarchy and score with the public, the AVP needs a boost... make that a jolt. And as a defibrillator helps shock a weary heart, so does the Olympic Games jack up attention in this game. Every four years, this supreme sports showcase attracts millions of casual American fans who drop everything to watch their country compete. For those who catch beach volleyball for the first time, they are amazed by how physically demanding the sport is. Sure the sand is soft, and the weather is warm. However, watching players racing around the court, diving towards dipping balls, jumping to forcefully serve, and leaping skyward for powerful spikes brings new meaning to the sport. Any former impressions these viewers had of the game – like lazily plopping the ball over the net with one hand while holding a beer in the other – quickly fade. "A lot of people change their tune, more men than women, when they come to an event and they realize it's not that easy to walk in the sand. And here we are running and jumping and they see the athleticism, so their tune changes," said Misty May-Treanor.

Nevertheless, this popularity windfall is simply not enough to carry Pro Beach Volleyball through the next Olympic Games quadrennial. The AVP cannot simply lie back and wait for an onrush of newly converted fans. Therefore, it understandably has relied on the media to court a larger fan base. "The name of the game is diversifying the way you get your content out," said Rich Feinberg, Vice President of Motorsports for ABC-ESPN.[4]

The AVP has trialed different outlets with varying degrees of success. First up, the print media. Try as it may, the AVP's public relations effort has steadily been plagued with problems in spreading the word. Error-laden press releases – sometimes retracted, sometimes not – have left many shaking their heads. For instance, announcements touting the inaugural Hot Winter Nights (HWN) 2008 indoor tour were incorrect and baffling. Luckily, a few experienced sportswriters correctly interpreted these misstatements and reformatted them into correct and understandable copy. But the majority of writers, who were unfamiliar with the sport, unknowingly propagated this misleading info in their HWN stories – not the publicity the AVP needed to kick off its new tour.

From the curious public's viewpoint, the AVP stands behind this dubious presentation of itself... way behind. Seldom do the tight-lipped executives, most with zilch for a beach volleyball background, readily reply to media inquiries, content to remain secluded in their Los Angeles office instead. When pressed, they respond with braggadocio and nonchalance, befitting a politician wriggling away from probing questions. Want some examples? Countering claims of low tournament turnouts, downplaying dismal relations with its players, and dismissing poor financial results are just a few.

To its credit, however, the AVP has made positive strides. First, it has partnered with a magazine, *DIG*, to promote itself and the players. Fortunately, this publication covers the AVP well. But it comes complete with numerous self-serving and sugar-coated stories, far removed from edgier and in-depth coverage in other publications about other sports. Second, keeping up with the times, the AVP in 2007 heavily invested in a new website, designed by Major League Baseball's (MLB) Advanced Media unit, to replace an outdated one that was disorganized and confusing. During the first year, the visitors raved about the user-friendly and visually stimulating site that provided tournament schedules, player profiles and photos, and the popular message board for fans to comment and vent about beach volleyball. Probably the most popular feature was Game Day Central, which allowed a sneak-peek inside the action on tournament weekends. Given its overriding goal of reeling in techno-savvy visitors, the AVP also streamed live videos of matches. Despite this popularity, especially among its targeted, young fan base, it pulled the plug on this feature in 2008 – presumably for cost-cutting reasons. In the court of public opinion, frustrated fans could only shake their heads in disbelief.

I Like to Watch

The AVP could only do so much on its own to attract fans, and its efforts were a mixed bag of success. By far, however, the most important media for any sports organization is television. Without it, a sport does not stand a chance of connecting with fans and, in turn, convincing sponsors to invest.

Looking back at the Sydney 2000 and Athens 2004 Olympic Games, NBC reported that international audience ratings for its prime time beach volleyball coverage were among the top for all events, just behind such faves as swimming and track and field – both coincidentally recognized for body-hugging uniforms as well. "We saw this as one of the hottest venues at the last two summer Olympics," said Jon Miller, NBC Sports Senior Vice President.[5] The sport is indeed tele-friendly with its compact court, simple rules, fit athletes, fast action, party scene, and of course, its sexy image. Most def, "Must See TV."

An officially published report confirmed that the players at the Athens Olympics were indeed specially highlighted on television.

"More than 20% of the camera shots were found to be tight shots of the women players' chests and just over 17% of the shots were coded as buttock shots which, it is argued, leaves viewers with lasting memories of players' bodies rather than of memories of athleticism." The study concluded, "Such analysis of the visual coverage of the games confirms that sex and sexuality were used to not only promote the athletes but to sell the sport to viewers around the world."[6] Once again, another corporate-funded study whose results could have been easily obtained by interviewing guys at a sports bar!

Given this Olympics interest, the AVP also sought a worldwide audience for its tournaments. By negotiating deals with overseas distributors like China's Guangdong Television, its outdoor events have reached millions of viewers in numerous countries. This source of income was small but steady, and the AVP needed to grab whatever revenue, and exposure, it could get.

Despite these television successes abroad, the AVP has constantly suffered on the domestic front. During the mid-1990s when the pro sport peaked, numerous tournaments were broadcast live by NBC each year. However, when the AVP failed to fill the commercial time slots with sponsor ads, NBC yanked the cord, citing "decreased fan interest," a polite cover for its frustration with AVP management during those turbulent years. As luck would have it, newcomer Fox Sports Network (FSN) stepped up to the serving line – well, sort of. In the late 1990s, it aired taped events, in select regions, sometimes weeks later, and often very late at night. At least Pro Beach Volleyball was getting some air time, albeit competing with infomercials and test patterns for groggy, night owl attention.

To fix this gloomy TV picture, the AVP had to bite the bullet to reconnect with NBC during its 2001 rebuilding year. The humbled

AVP staff had to acknowledge the wrongdoing of its former management and convince NBC to televise tournaments again. At the negotiating table, the desperate AVP folded its hand, conceding many of the rights that a typical sports property could assert. First, the AVP was required to pay broadcasting and programming fees to gain air time – a rare obligation among sports properties that typically receive rights fees as income from their broadcasters. Second, the AVP issued close to a million shares of its stock to NBC, in exchange for this coverage, as a barter of sorts.[7] Third, it assumed the routine broadcaster burden of filling advertising slots during the telecasts, and therefore had to pursue advertisers on its own. Faced with a "damned if I do, damned if I don't" dilemma, AVP management signed the one-sided contract. In beach volleyball terms, it was "getting domed."

"Once we set ourselves and our credibility, we have a place at NBC where we can grow. There's certainly the opportunity for us if we perform well," said the hopeful Armato.[8] The AVP knew it had to be patient in hopes the corporations' confidence and respect would be revived. For example, NBC agreed to show a whopping two tournaments in 2002, a far cry from its 1994 lineup of ten tournaments. Because of the AVP's minimal leverage and the sport's shaky popularity, it was not unusual for these shows to be cut up, shortened, or even cancelled during the early 2000s by these broadcasters. Can you imagine watching the last play of a closely fought match and, all of a sudden, the screen blanks out and the closing credits are rolling? Don't laugh, it happened!

Don't Turn That Dial

However, on the heels of the U.S. medal wins by the four women in the Athens 2004 Olympics, fan interest in the sport increased and new agreements were reached not only with NBC but also with FSN and FOX. Still, while more events would be televised, the AVP was deemed "not worthy" and continued to give in to network demands. To save face and restore at least some dignity, the groveling AVP put a positive spin on a 2006 deal with FSN in carefully crafted press releases and financial statements. "Fox Sports *will contribute* the time and production of the event and *will receive* additional equity in AVP."[9] Translation: The AVP issued millions of shares of stock to FSN to compensate this company for 1) doing its own work and 2) the "privilege" of televising AVP events.

Fortunately, with its popularity growing into 2007, all 18 AVP event finals were televised, with certain tournaments watched by over one million households. Because of this momentum, FSN and NBC started to position these shows right after strong lead-ins (e.g., MLB, and the AST X-Games Dew Tour, respectively). Even better, the time slots for these Pro Beach Volleyball championship matches were expanded from one to two hours, in certain cases. Last, in seeking added exposure at season's end, the AVP contracted to have two tournaments nationally shown on the newcomer cable station, My Network TV.

So, instead of one big, fat television contract that other esteemed sports bank on, the AVP had to resort to a hodgepodge of broadcast options. Managing all these outlets has been a drain on its bottom line and the lean staff. By year's end, the optimistic AVP, whose confining contract with FSN had ended, began seeking partners to televise its HWN 2008 indoor tour, as well as its Crocs 2008 outdoor tour. "Now we are a free agent and we are going to look around and see what the opportunities are," said Armato.[10]

But despite beach volleyball's increased viewership in 2007, baseball, golf, and NASCAR summer audience ratings have been "roofing" those of the AVP by double or triple. Granted, Pro Beach Volleyball is far from being a big league sport. However, shouldn't the AVP command more attention and respect than such televised sports as billiards, darts, and lumberjack contests? And why do old fat guys gambling at a poker table draw more viewers than young, slender hotties running around in the sand?

For many, it takes just one glimpse of Pro Beach Volleyball action to get hooked. For example, consider the several hundred million viewers of the Athens Olympics beach volleyball events who were left wanting more, and who eagerly await the Beijing 2008 Olympic Games. In the months leading up to the 2008 Olympics, NBC was once again salivating in expectation of record Olympic ratings. The AVP, as always, could only hope that this large-scale, addictive audience would also tune in to its televised tour events.

Yet the AVP is held hostage – by its own troublesome past that it constantly seeks to distance itself from, and by the networks that clearly have the upper hand. It needs cost-effective and prominent face time on TV to lure more fans to the sport. It must also parlay its popularity to leverage better television contracts, complete with fuller event coverage in additional markets. However, it faces a Catch-22. To tempt networks, it must not only prove it has an audience, it also must show that it has landed sufficient sponsorship backing to fill the commercial slots. Yet these corporate supporters will only contribute if they're assured their ads will get prominent television exposure. Consequently, the AVP, like other mid-level sports, is in a bind, and it needs all the help it can get.

Eight

GETTING THE MOST BANG FOR YOUR BUCK

As the television camera zoomed in on her well-tanned and well-toned butt, Rachel Wacholder was bent over – ready for the next play. The former part-time model and now elite player flickered her fingers just below her waistline. While careful not to obscure the vivid corporate logo emblazoned on her bright red bikini bottom, she flashed a secretive signal to her partner and the million television viewers. Just another value-added exposure for the appreciative AVP partner, Speedo.

Exposure like this is what corporate sponsors dream about. The AVP prides itself on these visual opportunities, the end product of all its well-orchestrated marketing, negotiation, and coordination work. Within an exceedingly crowded sports entertainment industry, it must scramble for every sponsorship dollar. Unfortunately, in lockstep with its own roller-coaster past, the AVP's track record in landing lucrative sponsor deals has been inconsistent and unreliable.

During the height of Pro Beach Volleyball in the 1990s, Miller Brewing Company was tapping into the AVP to the tune of $100 million as its primary sponsor.[1] And in the years leading up to the Atlanta 1996 Olympic Games, other sponsors rushed to sign up. Proctor & Gamble, Coca Cola, Honda, and Kodak were just a few who nabbed a bite out of this runaway success of a sport. Back then, everyone wanted a piece of the action as "The Official (Product Type) of the AVP." Of course, the player-run AVP organization welcomed these companies with open arms.

In return for their million dollar payments, the sponsors, naturally, expected to be treated with respect. However, according to Mike Dodd, "The young AVP players felt that they didn't need to do anything extra to promote the sport. They often did not meet sponsor demands in exchange for support." When the sponsors saw their corporate money used to stoke tournament prize money instead of promoting their products in TV commercials or at tournaments, they were enraged. Adding insult to injury, some players demonstrated this "gimme the money" mentality on a more personal level during sponsor promotional events. "Miller kept the league afloat for many years and the sponsor reps would go into a bar and the players would be in there drinking Bud," said Steve Vanderpool, public relations counsel for Miller's AVP sponsorship.[2] Worse, complaints from these now agitated sponsors were all but ignored. Angry that their funding had been wasted, companies including Miller Brewing Company, Proctor & Gamble, and Honda took their loot and ran from this organization they now labeled as "damaged goods." So that by 1999, only a few loyal sponsors remained committed to the AVP.

A New Mission

When Leonard Armato took over the helm in 2001, he faced an up-hill battle to regain lost sponsor income. The country was tumbling into a recession, and sponsor advertising budgets were tightening. What would normally be an easy sell to sponsors – action, beach, and sex – proved to be extremely difficult.

To combat this negative perception, the resolute Armato pur-sued a threefold mission: resurrecting alliances with those spon-sors that bailed in frustration, reassuring those few that hung on during the bankruptcy years, and reaching out to new companies. Unfortunately, attempts to first reconnect with those who left were the equivalent of an unsuccessful plea bargain. Sponsors could not be coaxed to come back, having long closed the door on the AVP. However, he did rekindle damaged alliances with the companies still hanging in there – albeit by a net thread. For example, Wilson Sporting Goods and Paul Mitchell continued their sponsorships during the AVP downfall when fan interest was at an all-time low. To allay their fears of being mistreated and ignored again, he cajoled these corporations who welcomed these reassurances. Julie Sol-wold, Vice-President-Sports Marketing at Paul Mitchell, said, "The sport needed someone with vision, finances, and passion. There has been passion as long as I can remember, but there haven't been the business connections, and Leonard can open doors that couldn't be opened before."[3] However, Armato's biggest task, by far, was to court new sponsors by peddling a brand-new AVP – one much more attuned to and respectful of its clients. He lobbied these firms with assurances that they would be cared for and would receive value for their expenditures. Of course, flashing new player con-tracts, whose clauses now required strict allegiance to sponsors, was a plus. "The expectations are high for the AVP this time around.

What they are doing is what they should have been doing all along – protecting the sponsors," said Jim Andrews, Editorial Director at the IEG sponsorship consulting firm.[4]

Of course, these corporations are always striving to get the most bang for their buck, and investing in Pro Beach Volleyball versus other sports is a big decision. They require affirmation that their return on investment goals will be achieved, and that they will be protected. During sponsor negotiations over the next several years, the strong-handed Armato comforted the wary sponsors by issuing such forceful statements as "We control every aspect of our sport in a way that's unlike any other sport. We control the promotion, the publicity, what the players wear, the broadcasts, and the venues that we build from scratch so we can integrate our sponsors organically into them and into our TV production."[5] The sales pitch this time around was easier than in the past, due to the added bonus of women players now competing on the tour. Bruce Binkow, AVP Chief Marketing Officer, said, "It's all part of the sex appeal of the event, which can leave fans in the crowd fixated. It's fantastic on television, and it's absolutely captivating on-site."[6]

To lure cautious sponsors even closer, the desperate AVP has relied on outdated and questionable studies to measure the benefits of sponsorship. First, the AVP has continually asserted that it is the fastest growing U.S. sport in terms of fans. To support this claim, it dusts off a dated study conducted by a sports marketing firm that issues reports like these for a price.[7] Second, while relying on another consultant's research and its own records, the AVP has continually reported that its annual fan attendance has exceeded one million.[8] This unsupported milestone figure is still smugly stated in various press releases, financial statements, and at sponsor meetings to tout the tour's popularity. Take, for example, the 2007 season with its 18 three-day tournaments. By doing the math, approximately 20,000 fans would have attended each day – a highly suspect figure considering the average main stadium capacity is just a few thousand seats. But, that's their story and they're sticking to it. According to Armato, "Sponsorship is the lifeblood of the AVP, so we take our relationships very seriously."[9] If some sponsors only knew....

Fortunately, Armato had yet another, stronger selling point for these sponsors – his successful branding of basketball star Shaquille O'Neal into a universal icon in such varied ways as commercials, movies, and music. He highlighted the use of O'Neal's well-marketed image to achieve his brand recognition. Similarly, by pitching an "integrated exposure" platform approach, he assured each sponsor of optimum visibility of both its logo and product at tournaments, on television, and even in print. "The fact that everything was in one package, from the TV to the on-site to the overall sponsorship, was great. So often in today's landscape, the rights are divided up," said Jeff Urban, a Gatorade sports marketing director.[10] Sponsors welcomed this cost-effective, one-stop-shopping approach, one that shifted the onus from them to the AVP to coordinate and manage this integration.

New Lifeblood – Drips at a Time

Recognizing these benefits, companies such as Gatorade, Bud Light, Microsoft's Xbox, and Nissan, which became the tour's title sponsor in 2003, were reeled in early on. These new sponsors were pleased that NBC had agreed to resume its coverage of AVP events so that their commercials could run in slots filled by the AVP. In contracts regularly ranging from a scant half-million to a relatively modest two million dollars, sponsors were assured of integrated product exposure through logos the players wear, tournament banners shown in competition footage, and airings of its TV commercials. On-site, the accommodating AVP set up sponsor signs and tents, complete with tables, displays, and interactive games for the fans. They further coordinated with television crews to ensure that the commercials would run as scheduled, and that the signage, as a backdrop to the finals event, would be seen by the TV viewer. The Nautica sportswear company, for one, has unendingly benefited from this partnership. To this day, at each tournament site, Nautica's colorful sponsor tent draws crowds for player autograph sessions, gift giveaways, and peeks at its latest clothing line. Also, its sailboat logo is noticeable as a tattoo on player arms or as an insignia on referee shirts. For each televised event, Nautica's court-bordering signs are clearly visible, sponsorship is reiterated by commentators, and sailing commercials are aired.

Recently, other blue chip corporations like McDonald's, Hilton Hotels, and Nature Valley Granola, have joined the ranks, towering over such newcomers as American Licorice and IZone sunglasses. As a new contract is signed, both the AVP and the sponsor jointly issue a press release that extols the virtues of the product and its fit with beach volleyball. This mutual back-scratching by sponsor marketers ("The AVP is a perfect match for...") and by the AVP management ("This sponsor clearly represents the fun and excitement of the beach lifestyle...") celebrates a new partnership with high hopes. They know the drill!

And a valued sponsor has even returned to the lineup. In a blast from the past, the Jose Cuervo Tequila company rejoined in 2006 after a ten-year hiatus. Cuervo was one of the AVP's oldest sponsors – advertising at tournaments in the AVP's first year, 1983. Back then, its three-story tall inflatable bottle flanked the courts, lazily teetering back and forth in the warm sea breezes. For sure, a hazy sign of the times and the laid-back vibe that Cuervo sought to snatch. But, by 1996, Cuervo too became disgruntled with the way it was treated and bolted. But how times have changed. Cuervo is now one of the hottest sponsors on tour, joining fellow booze sponsors Bud Light and Barefoot Wines. It is hopeful that the past beach volleyball spirit, of which it played a huge role in creating, will be revived. "We feel the AVP Tour has grown to the point where it can provide us with an even greater opportunity to reach our target consumers," said Bertha Gonzalez, Jose Cuervo Commercial Director.[11] Cuervo undoubtedly has the biggest on-site presence and has always been a fan favorite. Along sponsor row, at each 2007 event, flirtatious bikini models lured passersby to the "Cuervo Cabana" with its pulsing music, lounge chairs, and big-screen TVs where fans watched the AVP action. Nearby, a stand sold shots and mixed drinks. And rowdy beauty contests were held where males and females strutted their stuff in front of packed main stadium crowds who text-messaged votes for their favorites.

However, despite this influx, some sponsors have parted with the AVP. A few small minnows slipped through the AVP netting, giving it a go as either a short-term trial, or even as a gamble. For instance, the I-Joy Robotic Massage Chair with its pulsating vibrations, moved on after just one year of providing free massages at events. Also, Frank's Red Hot Sauce bit off more than it could chew with its "Battle to the Bone" chicken wing eating contests that pitted AVP pros against hungry fans. Last, after signing a multi-year contract to market its unique, interactive cell phone product geared to the Millennial crowd, the New Motion company's promising promotion flamed out in the first year. Fortunately, AVP management can live with these small-scale losses – realizing that there are more fish in the sea.

Unfortunately, many big catches have gotten away too. Long-time "umbrella sponsor" Nissan, whose company name blanketed AVP tour advertising for three years, did not renew its contract beyond 2005. Highly respected among the fans and players, Nissan initially claimed its company was "the perfect fit with the AVP." This company became the heir to the dominant Miller Brewing Company's AVP title throne of the 1990s. It held slot car races for fans, conducted raffles of its vehicles, and issued Xterra SUVs to the season's champions. Although its true reason for not renewing has never been publicized, many believe that Nissan abruptly left because it felt mistreated. The ambitious AVP, in an attempt to make more money off of other sponsors, downplayed Nissan's prominence. For example, within AVP advertisements promoting the tour, banners displayed: "Nissan Series, Boulder Open, sponsored by LIFTOFF." And the AVP's response to this departure? "They just didn't look like active sponsors that would advance the tour. So we thought it was time to move on," said Armato.[12]

The AVP promptly sought to fill this prized, top sponsor slot. Crocs, the unconventional footwear company, was on the prowl – seeking a wider market for its ultra-successful line of offbeat shoes. A promising partnership was soon forged. "We looked around and saw that the property had grown really quickly. It was kind of a risk when we first started last year (2006) but it worked out very well for us," said Crocs CEO Ron Snyder.[13] Tournament signage displaying the Crocs logos on welcome banners, volleyball nets, and court boundaries, suddenly became visible at every turn. And an oversized, inflatable Crocs shoe flanked the court on which it hosted clinics led by Sinjin Smith.

Big Gains and Losses

Crocs was soon selling close to 1,000 pairs of its lifestyle shoes each tournament, and crediting its phenomenal growth, in part, to its tie-in to the AVP tour. Shortly thereafter, Crocs signed a five-year, contract extension in 2007. This major commitment and multi-million dollar revenue, although small-scale compared to the former Miller Brewing Company sponsorship, was the shot in the arm the struggling AVP needed. As the 2008 tour approached, the new partners were venturing forward hand in hand, hoping that this symbiotic arrangement will lead to long-term prominence.

For without sponsorship dollars, the AVP would be history. To survive, it must continually rely on this huge revenue source, approximating 85 percent of its income each year. This income stream has fortunately grown from $6 million in 2003 to $19 million in 2007, when the busy AVP painstakingly managed uniquely tailored contracts for over 20 national and regional sponsors.

But what shocked many observers was the exodus of so many sponsors leading up to the 2008 season. Despite the Beijing 2008 Olympic Games wave that will bring more attention to the sport, 30 percent of the sponsors did not return. To be sure, companies like American Licorice, IZone, and SolarSafe will not be missed. However, the pullouts by such majors as Microsoft, Schick, Herbalife, and Jet Blue severely impacted AVP's precarious bottom line by millions of dollars. Rumors began to fly about the reasons for these departures... including the sponsors' dissatisfaction with AVP management and a perceived loss of investment value. Compounding this predicament, disgruntled AVP marketing executives also bolted in early 2008. Once again, at a critical point in its history, the AVP seemed to be shooting itself in the foot.

Withdrawals like these not only impact the AVP, but also the higher-ranked teams, among them Misty May-Treanor and Kerri Walsh. The AVP funnels prime sponsor endorsement deals to these players, like Wacholder, who receive payments for donning clothing, signing autographs, and appearing at promotions. But given Schick's and Jet Blue's absence, the elite-level athletes, Phil Dalhausser and Matt Fuerbringer, respectively, have lost a sizeable chunk of change, and will have to await another gifted handout.

But what about the vast majority, the remaining 90 percent of the players who are in most need of funds? They can only dream about these endorsement gold mines. Confined by even more restrictive contractual clauses, often subject to off-the-cuff and questionable interpretation by the AVP, they are constrained as they seek sponsorships and publicity – even on their own. This scenario is far from ideal, for the AVP cannot survive without its players. And these players, if they want to succeed in this sport, cannot survive without the AVP.

Nine

SURVIVAL OF THE FITTEST

"Is it normal to live off of Top Ramen and sleep on friends' couches to pursue one's dream? Maybe it comes down to the fact that we just need to know that if we work hard enough, someday it (financial security) will be there for us too," said Hans Stolfus, a middle-ranked journeyman on the AVP tour.[1]

As the sole professional beach volleyball organization in the United States, the AVP tour is the primary vehicle for players to earn a living by playing the game they love. The AVP realizes it has no tour without these players, but the vast majority of these athletes don't feel cared for or cared about. They face so many challenges, far more than the top athletes in other professional sports, that many continually question whether they can stick it out.

Competing in one of the top beach volleyball tours in the world, the AVP players are among the best... anywhere. Approximately 200 contracted athletes compete in the AVP, ranging in age from the upper teens into the forties. Pro Beach Volleyball, on the fringe of mainstream sports, attracts a unique type of player – a maverick of sorts. These non-conformists, who are tired of the indoor competition, transition to the beach – in effect, learning to excel at a whole new game. For example, Stolfus made the move to the beach game in 2001 after competing at San Diego State University. These competitors are drawn to this unique sport, complete with the fun-loving lifestyle, free-spirited vibe, and no-holds-barred play. As a throwback to the game's roots, bravado runs rampant through the ranks because tackling these new challenges requires a certain courtside confidence.

Overall, they're a close-knit posse. Although there are computer-calculated ratings, no stigmatizing class system exists within the player ranks. No marking of territories. No erecting of fences. Each player is genuinely supportive of the other, whether offering sideline encouragement during matches, splitting travel expenses, sharing sponsorship leads, or even suggesting strategies or new skills that, when honed, could be potentially used against them. So, it is this special camaraderie that best defines this community, that serves as the backbone of support, and that now unifies this new "Association" of Volleyball Professionals. A mirror of the extremely tight alliance that founded the AVP twenty-five years ago to safeguard player rights.

The Ties That Bind

The current AVP organization is a monopoly. No ifs, ands, or buts. Whether it likes to admit it or not, it has a stranglehold on the players who compete in its tournaments. The AVP requires these "independent contractors" (who meet certain qualifying criteria) to sign a contract, aka "Player Agreement." Although the binding legality of this document can be questioned, this captive clientele can only earn money by signing it. The AVP has an upper hand, needless to say, and the approximate 200 players must endure such restrictions within the 2005 four-year contract that:[2]

> ➤ Specify the prize money that can be earned,

> ➤ Limit their missing of tournaments to certain conditions,

> ➤ Punish them for unsportsmanlike conduct,

> ➤ Relinquish their licensing rights as players to the AVP for its commercial use, and

> ➤ Prevent them from contracting with sponsors who compete with AVP sponsors.

These five imposing clauses have come back to haunt the AVP in so many unsuspecting ways.

First, unlike other professional sports, all Pro Beach Volleyball players, regardless of their ranking, are not guaranteed any salary. Per the contract they sign, these ballers only get paid on a "per-tournament" basis, contingent on their performance. This arrangement is similar to the pro tennis and golf tours where players earn money based on their tournament results. However, the AVP athletes earn peanuts compared to these counterparts. For instance, a single weekend's PGA purse typically exceeds an entire year of AVP multi-million dollar prize money! At the individual level, a typical PGA winner in 2007 earned several hundred thousand dollars for a weekend's play. Compare that to a first place AVP athlete in 2007 who earned no more $15,000. Furthermore, the PGA tour ordinarily pays out tens of thousands at the 32nd place level; whereas the AVP pays out only a few hundred bucks at this last money-earning tournament finish spot. Overall, only the top 24 athletes (the top six elite men's and women's teams) are estimated to earn enough prize money and sponsor revenue to comfortably make a living each year. For the remaining 90 percent – the have-nots – most struggle to get by on earnings well below the annual poverty level of $10,787.[3] Dozens of teams bring home nada, not even a T-shirt, each and every tournament. Even Logan Tom, a one-time rising star who has since left the tour, said, "There's no money on the beach. It is something you do mainly because you enjoy doing it."[4]

Earnings are one thing, but what about player expenses? "Each player is responsible for his or her own housing and travel to and from events," reads the contract clause that stirs discontent in the ranks. Players know full well that, in other major professional sports, all travel expenses are absorbed by the team owners or the league. Therefore, on an ordinary AVP event weekend, an amazing two-thirds of the players lose out. They have to cover airfare, food, lodging, and car rental – all of which offset their meager earnings. Although these travel expenses vary depending on the location and how far a player advances into the event, these weekend expenses can easily reach $1,000. For a typical tournament in 2007, only the top 16 men's and women's teams earned enough to cover travel expenses, using this rule of thumb. "We're competing for a limited amount of prize money. We travel so much that it is important to make enough money to at least break even.... which is tough when the level of competition increases each year," said middle-ranked Angie Akers.[5] To shave costs, many players resort to sleeping on floors of low- or no-star hotel rooms, surviving on fast food, and sharing overcrowded rental cars. There are also unconfirmed, urban legends of guys waking up in the beds of groupies – a self-effacing, yet cost-cutting measure! Using this criterion, Stolfus was fortunately in the black, earning over $25,000 in 2007. But when other expenses such as coaching, training, equipment, and clothing (custom-fitted bikinis can cost a few hundred bucks alone) are included, only the few elite teams can cover these costs by relying on prize money alone.

Second, many players are prohibited from missing a tournament to compete on another tour. The punishment for a "no-show" takes many forms. But there are exceptions to every rule. And the AVP has applied this axiom time and time again in its tailored contracts with the elite athletes at the "head of the class." However, when these stars break contract rules, the AVP must respond on the fly. Just like a teacher handles an unruly student while maintaining order in the class, the AVP faced this scenario midway through the 2007 tour. Who would have guessed that the AVP's cherished Golden Goddesses, Misty May-Treanor and Kerri Walsh, would test management's patience and challenge its control? Sure enough, in pursuit of their Olympic dreams, they played hookey by skipping a July AVP event in Seaside Heights, New Jersey to compete in an Olympic-qualifying Federation Internationale de Volleyball (FIVB) tournament in Montreal. Their absence alarmed many: sponsors, fans, fellow players, and even the AVP executives. Management quickly convened to decide how to best handle this truancy. They faced a few alternatives: scold the pair, ignore their transgression, or bend the rules to appease their now fuming competitors. While considering these options, they realized the duo's actions were in the best interest of the sport. As a result, they caved-in and permitted this absence. Then, to quell the uproar among the players, the AVP saved face and announced a "dispensation plan" to excuse other elite Olympic-aspiring teams, from certain AVP events – the equivalent of a hall pass.

Third, the AVP contract dictated unisex rules for on-court behavior, a sharp contrast to the 1980s and 1990s, when tantrums and antics by the volleyball gods were not only permitted, but lauded. Back then, heated rivalries between such pairs as Tim Hovland/ Mike Dodd and Randy Stoklos/Sinjin Smith were commonplace. The taunting of opponents and referees, practically taboo now, became accepted as part of the show. Whether it was pulling down nets, throwing out second-place awards, or mooning referees, all these actions were pure entertainment for the fans.

Nowadays, while considering contract penalties for unsportsman-like behavior, the guys have necessarily adopted a kinder, gentler persona. Not wanting to break restrictive sportsmanship contract rules nor rile potential sponsors, players today are often politically correct, toeing the corporate line. Hell, even a polite golf clap after a play is a stretch for some! Certainly, there are no bad boys who are the equivalents of their sports' forefathers, and certainly no John McEnroe or Terrell Owens wannabes. Nor can any men claim even a fraction of the fame that Derek Jeter or Lebron James has earned. The only player who has come close to grabbing such positive public attention was three-time Olympic medalist Karch Kiraly, and he retired at the end of the 2007 season. Clearly, this AVP vice grip has curbed the male showmanship instinct. Even the 6'9" Phil Dalhausser, an elite player who is changing the game by his dominating presence and prowess, cannot be tapped. Off the court, he is politely reserved – not quite the spokesperson the AVP so desperately needs.

Fourth, the AVP certainly owns these athletes. According to the contract, the AVP gets paid when the player's "likeness" is used by its sponsors.[6] The athletes are handcuffed, and at the AVP's mercy, for their images can only be promoted by the AVP. "They've got to get these players out in the mainstream, whether it's aligning them with a major clothing line or charitable endeavor in the off-season," said Rob Jaynes, a former AVP marketing director.[7] Unfortunately, the financially strapped and minimally staffed AVP does not have the resources to properly blitz the media with player images and press releases to sell these players. It has enough trouble even promoting itself. "We have great athletes on the tour, and they should be recognized more than they are," said Sean Rosenthal, one of the tour's elite players.[8] But, without the AVP's support and promotion, sponsors simply do not want to take a chance on an unknown.

Yet with minimal effort, the AVP financially benefits by simply steering the sponsors toward the higher-ranked athletes, while meeting any request to provide details about a player's bio, ranking, and stats. A "You rub my back, I'll rub your back" kinda deal. The highly sought after endorsement income from the national sponsors is dished out to those fortunate few, who get first dibs on prized deals with such corporations as Speedo, Hilton Hotels, and Jose Cuervo Tequila.

In exchange, when players agree to wear tattoos, sign autographs, and appear in print ads or commercials, they help the sponsors grow brand recognition. Players are obliged to wear the sponsor's logo on their swimsuit, cap, or body – sometimes provocatively. The infatuating butt is a sure-bet sponsor billboard for the women, whose lower backs are branded with "tramp stamp" emblems and whose bikini bottoms are embroidered with corporate imprints. One Olympic hopeful, Jennifer Boss, wears "RO" on one cup and "XY" on the other in support of this swimsuit company. But even though the women have the anatomical edge in terms of options, the men's board shorts and shoulder sides also advertise sponsor product designs and names. For instance, an elite-level pair, Mike Lambert and Stein Metzger, has been jokingly called "Team Nascar" by their jealous peers for all their visible endorsement deals. In any case, both on and off the court, players are mindful of their commitments, because on-site sponsor reps are always checking that their products are gaining visibility. "The key is to show the sponsors that we are helping their company get noticed and giving them good advertisement," said Matt Fuerbringer who toed the corporate line while wearing his Jet Blue cap proudly.[9]

Certain player endorsement contracts are the bomb, reaching the seven-figure mark – exceeding their annual prize money by several hundred thousand dollars. The Golden Girls, May-Treanor and Walsh, have the pick of the sponsor crop and rely on their agents to negotiate sweet, "nectar" deals with the likes of Gatorade and Nautica. In fact, they have been known to actually turn down requests, much to the amazement, and frustration, of their peers.

Also, pure good looks go a long way in securing sponsor deals. Team Gorgeous, Suzanne Stonebarger and Michelle More, has parlayed beauty into cool deals with AVP sponsors Jose Cuervo Tequila and Fiji Water. On their website, clearly geared towards sponsors, they flaunt their assets in teasing images both on and off the court, and openly offer such services as wearing company logos (on apparel or as tattoos) and making appearances at private events. Thanks to this branding, Team Gorgeous has enjoyed near-celebrity status by attending corporate parties, traveling overseas, and so on – benefits most teams salivate over. "It's been amazing so far to be able to make a career out of this," said Michelle More.[10] Many wonder if she's referring to her beach volleyball play or her endorsement contracts!

Fifth, players are restricted from signing with certain sponsors who are in direct competition with the AVP national sponsors. According to the AVP contracts with these companies, the AVP protects them by ensuring there will be no conflicts. For example, Coca Cola's Powerade is off limits to these players due to the AVP partnership with Gatorade. However, exceptions to these rules have been made, especially for the privileged few. Case in point, both

Todd Rogers and Rosenthal were issued the green light to be sponsored by two energy drink companies, Red Bull and Rockstar, respectively. Each of these athletes, among the best in the world, was often seen wearing clothing that promoted these products during AVP events in 2007. The twist here is that the AVP sponsor, Herbalife, marketed its own energy drink, Liftoff, at these same events. Therefore, who is in control of whom? And what kind of sponsor protection is this? It's no wonder that Herbalife ended its sponsorship in 2008, and the AVP took a hit to its financial pocket.

Scraping for Every Dollar

And so the story goes. The rich get richer, and the poor get poorer. What can the remaining majority, the lower- and middle-ranked contracted players do? Without the luxury of being handed sponsorships and without the stardom to negotiate favorable contracts with the AVP, they're on their own to scramble for extra income. These disadvantaged athletes need to independently and creatively market themselves, and this effort is quite time consuming.

For starters, several dozen players have created Internet websites, MySpace pages, and/or Facebook accounts. These latter two options – laced with bios, pictures, and videos – are more apt to be used for socializing than selling. For instance, Stolfus has only used MySpace, and minimally mentions his AVP career. As an exception, however, Alicia Polzin (26th-ranked on the 2007 tour) has been the most enterprising of all, advertising "Sponsors Wanted" as her eye-catching MySpace headline.

Still, these needy players must pursue sponsors in the traditional manner by beating down doors, making phone calls, and meeting with company representatives, ideally before the season starts and their travel expenses accumulate. In support, fellow AVP player and graphics designer Angela Lewis has assisted players create promotional portfolios to present to these companies.

They needed all the help they can get because, for many, a salesman's hat is ill-fitting. Players like Stolfus have trouble landing any deals, let alone those that the AVP will agree to. Some mid-level players, who wish to remain anonymous for fear of reprisal, complain that requests for sponsor approvals are often rejected by the AVP without logical or consistent reasoning. As a result, they must often resort to arrangements landed with local firms, or with friends who can swing deals with their employers. Of course, this income barely covers a small percentage of their expenses. But these desperate players will take all the scratch they can get from the likes of Olyos Pizza, Syzmo energy drink, and Tsunami Sushi – well off the mainstream, corporate path. Compounding this quest further, some of these sponsors only agree to provide support based on how the players do in competition. For example, if a team does not consistently place in the top ten, fuhgeddaboutit!

In desperation, some risk-taking players wear unapproved sponsor clothing, just like kids pushing their parents' buttons by challenging overly strict rules. But come on, does it really matter if an athlete is toting an Adidas backpack or warming up with a Powerade shirt? Apparently so, as evidenced by arguments between players and AVP management breaking out on the court. Repeated stories have been shared about hovering AVP executives who have swooped down on players during timeouts to reprimand them for wearing a shirt with an unauthorized corporate logo. If a player continually refuses to play ball, he can rule out even the smallest sponsor endorsement bone being thrown in his direction down the road. To justify the AVP stance, the dictatorial Armato said, "We must avoid the confusion in the marketplace and ensure that fans and sponsors get the AVP product they expect."[11] Yes sir!

United They Stand

So, what are the players doing about these contract restrictions that most all believe are injustices? For starters, many of them have taken out their frustration by smacking the official AVP ball that is adorned with Armato's signature. Yet others have been more constructive. Rallying together, these players – from the dirt poor to the millionaires – are bringing it on. Represented by a player's committee in the last few years, they have endlessly voiced their complaints to management. But recently they have upped the ante. In 2007, a Professional Beach Volleyball Association (PBVA), a conceivable forerunner to an eventual union, was formed with most all players joining. Initiated by a few athletes, among them a middle-ranked Jason Ring, this organization is standing up for player rights and challenging the hierarchy. Game on, AVP.

Of course, everyone likes a good feud. With the player contract up for renewal in 2009, this collective will challenge the terms in the new four-year contract. Their agenda of mandates for the AVP includes increasing prize money, easing restrictions on playing in other tours including Olympic-qualifying, sharing of licensing rights revenue, and relaxing sponsorship rules. What is amazing to many is that these "demands" match the benefits that athletes in other sports have been routinely enjoying for years.

Needless to say, the AVP is not a happy camper. It has dismissed any mention made of this upstart, yet potentially powerful organization. Against his will, Armato is faced with returning to his roots, having participated in the hauntingly similar player revolt that led to the 1983 birth of the AVP. Gearing up for a contract negotiations battle, he has already issued politically posturing statements, seeking to gain some sympathy. "We would love to give more prize money but we're limited in how much we can distribute. They have to understand that it takes perseverance and sacrifice. They have to love the game and the lifestyle," rationalized Armato.[12]

In any case, the generic contract will continue to be tailored, especially for the higher-ranked players whom the AVP most benefits from. In these cases, certain contract restrictions are relaxed to allow those with money to make even more money. This purposeful AVP divide-and-conquer strategy separates the haves from the have-nots. Through this preferential treatment, the AVP caters to these stars that draw the crowds.

This leaves the remaining players feeling like they're getting tooled. However, they reluctantly agree to these terms, complete with contract termination clauses for noncompliance. What else can they do? The players have long complained about such contract clauses but they face a "damned if I grumble, damned if I don't" scenario. Armato's well-worn and tattered motto, "We will always explore ways that our lower-ranked players can avail themselves of more benefits and opportunity" is long on optimism but short on practicality.[13] As a result, it simply falls on deaf ears.

Digging Deep

But these players cannot wait for management to man-up. These up-and-comers are determined to make a go at the sport they love. For instance, the 32nd-ranked Chrissie Zartman, has confidently hired an agent to help her seek sponsor dollars. But realizing that she might not be successful, "I am looking for a job that will give me the flexibility to train and play volleyball."[14]

Even when players are willing to moonlight with another job, they face an added dilemma. For instance, they need to devote substantial time to training and practicing to better compete and move up in the tour ranks. However, this commitment is not without its cost because they also must financially make ends meet. And that means holding down jobs to pay not only for living expenses but to cover these preparation costs. Of course, time spent working is time not spent readying for competition. Therefore, it's a no-win situation for most, and a prolonged trek to greatness for the fortunate few. The sympathizing Misty May-Treanor said, "It would be nice to have enough support behind our sport so that people who wanted to play wouldn't have to worry about a second job. They could do this and know they're going to make enough money to be all right."[15]

That's a pipe dream for sure, especially for so many financially-strapped athletes who must hold jobs year-round – ideally ones that are flexible enough to allow them to take off work for a few days to compete each weekend. Occupations like freelance journalists, part-time salesmen, real estate agents, graphic artists, and substitute teachers seem to be good, although not high-paying, matches. For instance, Stolfus writes a column for *DIG* magazine. Also, Tracy Lindquist, who works as a substitute teacher, slips in training when she can with her older sister and teammate Katie – often hitting the gym before the school day, and practicing on the beach at night. "If I could play full-time the way the top moneymakers could, that would be awesome. It's just not a possibility right now. I need the money to survive," she lamented.[16]

Compounding these job troubles is the high cost of living in the Los Angeles area, where most players reside year round. Kevin Cleary, who earned just $5,000 during his career, reflected, "When I started playing in the 1970s and 1980s, you could buy a house in the South Bay on a teacher's salary. I knew guys who would work 5, 6, 7 months and get by."[17] But times have certainly changed. Nowadays the off-season is minimal, and players can't rely on this autumn income to carry them through the rest of the year. "I have two weeks free in November, I have December and that's it. So, when people say, 'Oh, don't you just play in the summer?' Oh, no. It's a full-time job!" said the exasperated Boss.[18]

But players remain optimistic. "You always want to win a tournament, be in the top five and make money so you don't have to get a real job," said Nick Lucena, a 28-year-old who earned $38,000 in 2007 prize money.[19] Given the circumstances, young single players are best positioned to juggle their time and commitments. For them, it's a make-or-break proposition. Bearing minimal financial and family obligations, they're free to make a run for stardom. They recognize this opportunity won't last forever and they have the strength to work odd jobs, practice and work out at strange hours, and travel cross-country – all with no strings attached.

At the end of the day, Pro Beach Volleyball is a business. But it still is a sport and, theoretically, fun "Competing on the tour, for many, is simply a labor of love," said Carl Henkel, a fifth-place finisher at the Atlanta Olympics. But most all players face three strikes: minimal tournament earnings, limited sponsor income, and low-paying jobs. According to Mike Dodd, coach of Rosenthal, "The focus is always on competing, winning, making money, surviving, and trying to make it all work."[20]

Most live for the journey, not for the destination. But there comes a time when a player needs to decide what's more important: happiness or money. Tired of this grind, many realize that, after crunching the numbers, they cannot earn a living in this sport. They then drop out – often with high credit card bills in hand – leaving the sport well before reaching their potential and fulfilling their dreams.

But many continue to fight the good fight. These hopefuls will continue to reach for their goals while falling further into debt. "I'm broke as a joke," admits the struggling Stolfus, on the verge of a

2008 financial breakthrough, thanks to his silver medal finish at the Pan American 2007 Games.[21] Funny how a week at this "nonprofit" event has brought him and his partner, Ty Loomis, more notoriety and potentially a bigger income than six years on the financially crippled AVP tour.

Ten

TO HAVE AND TO HOLD?

"Marriage is popular because it combines the maximum of temptation with the maximum of opportunity." – George Bernard Shaw.

Close your eyes and imagine being with your perfect mate... to have and to hold; for better or for worse; for richer, for poorer; in sickness and in health; to love and to cherish from this day forward until death do us part.

Now wake up from your dream world, and welcome to the world of the AVP. Pro Beach Volleyball is a team sport... at least the last time we checked. Partners must rely on each other — on and, ideally, off the court. To succeed, both athletes on a team must click – physically, by extensive practicing, training, and competing; as well as mentally, by fostering rapport, trust, and commitment. Many players realistically estimate that three to four years are needed to gel. This period coincides with the timetable for the quadrennial Olympic Games, the pinnacle that players aspire to.

Kerri Walsh and Misty May-Treanor have proved that this model works. For seven years, they've mastered the game and personified the "team" ideal. Since first coupling in 2001, they have competed in over 125 tournaments. As the best beach volleyball team in the world, they have unarguably dominated the competition. Their long-lasting track record has positioned them for a likely second gold medal, this time at the Beijing 2008 Olympic Games, and has endeared them to long-term fans with the forming of the Mayniacs Fan Club, for instance.

"Kerri and I set goals and in order to meet those goals, you have to see progress," noted the pragmatic May-Treanor. "For us to stay at the top is very difficult because teams are getting better. We find ways to improve."[1] Despite this technical focus, they recognize that teamwork and camaraderie are vital. As Walsh said, "I absolutely love to play with Misty. We have come so far. I feel our partnership has grown every year."[2]

Shopping For A Partner

Other Pro Beach Volleyball teams can only dream of matching this pair's unparalleled success and longevity. But in reality, very few partners remain together longer than a season for they are always seeking a better match. While realizing it does take two, these independents are constantly looking out for number one. To them, there most certainly is an "I" in "Team." This cycle of breakups and hookups frustrates the AVP, which promotes the game as a team sport to cautious sponsors, wary media, and fickle fans who are often puzzled and frustrated by this constant churn.

"We always talk about partnerships being like marriages. When things are bad, you've got to figure out what's wrong and you've got to fix it. If you let problems go, they linger. If you don't get along, they'll show," said Eric Fonoimoana.[3] Therefore, finding the ideal partner is paramount. Everyone wants to win, and each player seeks a teammate to form the best match. Yet when compared to our society's divorce rate approximating 50 percent, the breakup rate among these pros is alarmingly higher.

In recent years, a vast majority of the approximate 200 contracted athletes has returned to the new AVP season with new teammates – hoping to take the tour by storm. Unfortunately, very few pairings have lasted beyond two seasons. Case in point, an alarming nine of the top ten men's teams in 2005 did not return together for the 2006 season... living and breathing an adapted version of an old adage: "If it ain't broke, fix it anyway."

As each new season starts, everyone curiously awaits this new look. Speculation runs rampant. *Did Justin get fed up with Gabe's injuries? Will Megan and Jessica pair up again, despite continually arguing last season? Will the tall rookie Max team up with the smaller veteran Steve?*

So what's going on behind the scenes, away from the curious public eye? Typically, during the off-season, each player reflects on the previous year's performance, sets goals for the next season(s), and decides whether his current partner will help reach them. And based on this assessment, choosing a new partner is practically a given.

That means almost everyone is searching for their best mate, and with such a huge pool of available competitors, the quest can be quite time consuming. The prime shopping season is winter, ideally a couple months before the season begins. Dain Blanton, Fonoimoana's gold medal partner, described the contacting process this way, "Most people have one another's phone numbers. You find out who you might be able to work with, and then if they are interested in playing with you."[4] E-mails are traded, text messages are sent, and phone calls are made to scope out an interest.

But, it's not as simple as it seems. Hidden from view, a certain pecking order dictates the matchmaking of partnerships. For starters, the elite competitors are not likely to seek a new partner, so these players are typically unavailable. At the start of the 2007 season, for example, the top three men's and top four women's teams remained together. Among them, of course, Walsh and May-Treanor returned as a unit after resolving, in the off-season, concerns even they had about their own communications. And fortunately so, because their Olympic Games goals require them to compete together in qualifying events stretching into July 2008. With this "Why ruin a good thing" philosophy, the top teams *usually* stick together... but not just for the prospect of an Olympic Team berth. Their prize money earnings and sponsor endorsement deals are the Cha-Ching that is music to their ears.

Because these elite-level pairings are set in stone, the remaining higher-ranked athletes use their standings as leverage to proposition others. In short, the player who is on top is the one in control; and those players next in line, who are seeking a new partner, would be foolish not to listen. For instance, Holly McPeak and Elaine Youngs parted soon after their 2004 bronze medal performance. As they sought new allies, each had the pick of the crop, commanding the attention of all other players.

"Complements in Order"

Of course, pairing up is a two-way street. Each player will want to partner with someone whose physique, skills, competitiveness, and even personality are in harmony with his own. The game of beach volleyball requires each partner to wear multiple hats. Yet only a few standouts on the tour have mastered all skills. Therefore, a player seeks an accomplice whose talents will help form a well-rounded twosome. Each player needs to serve, set, attack, and serve-receive, and the specialty skills of blocking and digging have been typically tied to a player's build. "It's like you choose your boyfriend or girlfriend. You gotta look – is one guy a blocker or a defender? You got to match up on paper skills wise, and know you're gonna get along with the partner too," said Mike Lambert who paired with his high school friend, Stein Metzger.[5]

Through its adoption in 2001 of the smaller court, the AVP has not only unintentionally and significantly altered the professional male and female player profile, but also caused a unique team-forming dynamic. This reduced playing area greatly benefits the taller player who can block more effectively with less terrain behind him, more successfully pound balls downwards despite the narrower court, and drill serves at wicked angles. These indoor "giants," traditionally not known for their quickness and mobility, soon infiltrated the ranks. For them, this simple change rocked, playing right into their large hands.

Yes, size does matter. Akin to other sports, height has also become a hot commodity in Pro Beach Volleyball. The athlete's demographic has gradually begun to change. During the early 2000s, very few men were taller than 6'5", and very few women taller than 6 feet. However, while the decade progressed, these tall players were highly sought after because of their commanding reach. The shorter, more experienced players took notice and began recruiting these newcomers, affectionately known as "big goofballs," due to their beach inexperience, clumsiness, and naïveté. Looking back, Karch Kiraly said, "In the past, it was, 'What ball-control player can I latch onto?' Now it's, 'What intimidator at the net can I latch onto?'"[6]

Therefore, in recent years, the team-forming "Tall-Short" strategy has successfully emerged, pairing a smaller, quicker defensive player with a tall, dominating tall player who can snuff out opponents' attacks through blocking. The classic example, of course, was when the 5'9" May-Treanor invited an apprehensive Walsh, a newcomer to beach volleyball, to be her partner. Looking back, Walsh said, "My learning curve personally wasn't as fast as I wanted it to be. Misty was really patient with me and worked through some of the most difficult times I have ever had in my career."[7] And before the 2006 season, the top-ranked, 6'2" Todd Rogers recognized his *shortcoming* as an *average-sized player* and sought out a tall cohort in his bid for the Beijing 2008 Olympic Games! A relative newcomer to the sport, the 6'9" Phil Dalhausser (aka "The Thin Beast") answered the call. In short order, this new pair also became a strong bet for a Beijing 2008 Olympic Games podium finish.

Apart from the blended physical traits, personalities need to mesh too. Is it critical for players to like each other? "It certainly helps to be able to get along well with your partner, but it's not a prerequisite," said the good-natured Kiraly, who won the gold medal at the Atlanta Olympic Games while competing with "Bad Boy" Kent Steffes. "I've seen partners who don't get along very well and don't socialize but still do great."[8] During the free-for-all 1990s, many guys competed just for the money – without a care about compatibility. For the sake of a common goal, they got along.

On the other hand, teammates with contrasting personas do thrive on and off the court. For example, a high-strung athlete often does well with a laid-back partner who keeps her from going off the deep end. And the easygoing player may need a kick in the butt at times from her more aggressive partner. Therefore, this opposites-attract formation it is well suited for these teams. Take, for example, the elite and extremely close team of Jenny Johnson Jordan and Annett Davis that has competed since 1997 – a current longevity record on the tour. According to Davis, "I am mellow and relaxed while Jenny is a fiery competitor."[9] The outgoing Jordan will often unleash her emotions on the court and argue a referee's call, charging up herself as well as Davis in the process. Whereas the reserved Davis's calming influence can settle down Johnson Jordan in time for the next play.

Yet, certain players are comfortable competing with a twin – someone who shares the same training and practicing beliefs, and who has a similar competitive drive. Of course, teammates can't get much closer than the sister act that competes on the tour. Katie and Tracy Lindquist have been continually playing together for eight years, and are ranked among the top 15 teams on the AVP 2008 tour. Watching the Lindquists is like watching Venus and Serena Williams play tennis doubles – you can see the teamwork and kinship bubbling over on the court. As the shortest team on the beach

(each stands at 5'6"), the siblings are well known for crafty defense and ball placement. Seldom does either block at the net, content to hang back and scoop up whatever comes their way. Their sisterly love and friendship makes it easy for them to compete. Despite the prospect of achieving more success by pairing up with a taller player, Katie dismisses this suggestion, "We play for fun. If we saw winning as our main goal, we would have to split up."[10]

In any case, once this courting is complete, players agree to form a team that is sometimes simply sealed with a handshake or hug. When they begin their preseason training, it can become quite clear during the early stages of dating whether or not they can make it last. What looked good on paper may not work in practice. Work ethics, playing strategies, and communication styles all need to be quickly evaluated by each player and jointly discussed.

Give-and-Take

Assuming both new partners agree to stick together, a higher level of commitment is needed. During these formative weeks, each is striving to make the partnership work – to prepare for the lengthy, six-month outdoor season, and beyond. Flexibility, understanding, and patience are critical, for how a player competed with a former partner may not work this time around. For instance, a player routinely prefers to play on either the left or right side of the court. If these two athletes favor the same side, one will need to change. A give-and-take approach soon develops, and negotiation is needed, just as in relationships when "which side of the bed" compromises need to be made. "If both players are willing to take the advice and criticism of the other, things can work out well," said John Hyden, an elite-level player.[11]

The game is personal – just you and your partner. The duo that gets along, shares common goals, and communicates well will consistently do better in the win column. Just like in everyday relationships, the couple shares their likes and dislikes, expressing preferences for sets and attacks, for example. Through this openness, they begin to connect and cooperate more, leading to improved play. Soon, the players are speaking the same language and are well on the road to potential glory.

As they solidify their alliance, one teammate may take on more of a coaching role. For example, because the giants have recently joined the tour, the smaller and typically more experienced ally has served as a mentor of sorts. The tall player, with her specialized net skills, usually requires a considerable amount of coaching to master all facets of the demanding beach game. Each "player-coach" must devote a lot of time and energy to teach, often at the expense of improving her own game. After her 2004 Olympic bronze medal, the no-nonsense, 5'7" Holly McPeak adopted this role by mentoring three taller partners through 2007. In what many call a "Camp Holly" stint, these newcomers learned about the entire game in what more closely resembled a boot camp, rather than summer camp. Even though McPeak's blocking days are history, she relied on her former net play experience to persistently teach Jennifer Boss, Nicole Branagh and Logan Tom about these front-row skills through regimented practices.

No matter how teams form, the proof of a partnership comes at game time. Hours of preseason drills and scrimmages can only carry the allies so far. The real payoff is at tournaments when competition is at its keenest and money is on the line. That's when the true player emerges, one who can step up and compete with her partner, while fighting for each and every point.

When the season begins, there are always high hopes for top finishes and sizeable payouts. During this honeymoon period, when all is rosy, the new bedfellows optimistically lavish praise on each other.

A Frustrated Counselor

Holly McPeak has single-handedly improved the women's game immeasurably as a player-coach. No other player in recent AVP history has invested as much time in teaching beach newcomers. Yet, her students have constantly pulled up their tent stakes and left Camp Holly. Here are snapshots of three protégés she has guided, and her candid views about these temporary partnerships.

For 2005, Jennifer Boss competed with McPeak for the entire season that culminated in a fifth-place ranking, up four notches from 2004. Boss then left McPeak to compete with Rachel Wacholder. "I love challenges and I love the hard work involved in getting a player to the level where she can win," McPeak said matter-of-factly.[26]

During 2006, Nicole Branagh, named the Most Improved Player-2006, competed with McPeak for most of the season before answering Elaine Youngs's call. McPeak's reaction? "My whole thing is developing young players. That (Branagh's departure) was disappointing, because you put so much time and energy into the partnership."[27]

In 2007, U.S. Olympic Indoor Volleyball Team phenom Logan Tom began the season with McPeak and her end-of-year ranking rose to thirteenth-place (from 40th place in 2006). At the season's start, the hopeful McPeak remarked about Tom, "She's a phenomenal athlete. We're aiming for the top."[28] Then, by mid-July, the frustrated McPeak ended this partnership, announced her 2008 retirement, and said, "We hit a wall and we weren't getting any better, and then our communications broke down. When I tried to fix it, things kept getting worse and worse."[29]

At the start of the 2005 campaign, for instance, the hopeful Youngs praised her new partner, a reserved Rachel Wacholder, "Rachel is easy to play with. It's a delight."[12] Although apprehensive at the start, Wacholder reciprocated, "Elaine has been great for me. She's patient with me."[13] Little did they know....

Understandably, duos that are consistently winning on the tour have figured out what works. They have invested much time, played in dozens of tournaments over the years, and developed a comfortable bond that will carry them further. These companions have learned each other's on-court strengths and weaknesses, likes and dislikes. They appreciate even more the traits of a successful partnership: intimidating offense, unrelenting defense, mental toughness, superb teamwork, strong competitive drive, and open communication.

In an ideal world, players make well-rounded decisions to form partnerships, flexibly accommodate their teammates, and persevere through all the ups and downs. However, most all beach volleyball pairings are just not meant to be. Call it boredom, call it impatience, call it ambition. All it takes is for one or both partners to get disillusioned. And this dissatisfied player, keeping all options open, competes for the moment with her teammate, while sneaking peeks for a new partner behind her back. During matches, she is not only sizing up her opponents but also checking out potential partners – always on the lookout for the perfect match. "Ninety percent of my partner changes have been my choice. In the past it was about positioning and playing with someone who could show me the way," admitted the driven, 28th-ranked Nancy Mason, during the twilight of her career.[14]

Breaking Up Is Easy To Do

Each season, dozens of partners divorce in a variety of ways, further chipping away at this team sport's foundation. The most civil option is for the pair to openly discuss concerns and, through a meeting of the minds, a decision is made to amicably part. "A lot of times it's agreed upon because sometimes you're not playing well and having poor finishes on a consistent basis. You say to each other 'Let's mix it up and try playing with other guys'," said Metzger.[15] As an example of an amicable separation, long-term partners and close friends 6'3" Casey Jennings and 6'8" Matt Fuerbringer discussed their 2007 season goals and recognized that a breakup would benefit both. The announcement of their split caught the entire volleyball community off-guard. "We wanted to be the best and we felt like we needed to step back and reevaluate our games individually with other guys," explained Jennings.[16]

A one-sided split can indeed be handled with grace and professionalism. For example, with regret, Dalhausser ended his 13th-ranked 2005 partnership with long-time friend Nick Lucena to compete with Rogers. "We were buddies. It was kind of awkward. I didn't like doing it at all, but for me it was a smart business decision," said the retrospective Dalhausser, top-ranked in 2007.[17] To this day, Lucena has never objected to his buddy leaving, because his ranking has also increased while competing with other partners.

Sadly, many split-ups are deviously and single-handedly masterminded. Rather than communicate face to face, the conniving player may start venting to others about his partner's play – in short, throwing his teammate under the bus. Then, seeking the warmth of a new bed, this cheater secretively begins to contact others. Stealthy phone calls or e-mails to potential partners lead to undercover practices held at obscure beaches. Before you know it, another pair of cohorts emerges. Sometimes this dumper will inform the dumpee – albeit by a sterile text message or e-mail. In a rare case, Metzger only found out about his partner Kevin Wong's departure after reading about it in the newspaper, at the same time as thousands of subscribers. "It was ugly as it gets," jabbed Metzger.[18]

Regardless of how the breakup unfolds, as the dumper moves onward, the dumpee is left behind in the cold. "It feels like the rug has been pulled out from under you," said Angie Akers, a veteran of nine AVP partnerships in seven years.[19] The deserted player, now a free agent, needs to pick up the pieces quickly. She must scramble to find another playmate, sometimes with just a day or two before the next tournament, and with no time to practice.

Often the juicy details of these clandestine breakups go unpublicized, with each player refusing to comment. The new team formations seemingly surface out of the blue, and puzzled fans are left to wonder what happened to their favorite team. However, in the case of the Boss/Wacholder tandem, each went public and put her own spin on their separation. Tit-for-tat barbs were exchanged. Wacholder said, "With the Olympics being very important to us, we thought we might be stronger with other people." Boss rebutted, "She dumped me. She thought I didn't have the heart and that I wasn't in good enough shape. I definitely have the heart for this and I'm definitely in shape."[20] Since then, each has found a new mate to make a run for a berth on the U.S. 2008 Olympic Beach Volleyball team.

In other cases, the divorce can get ugly, playing out like a soap opera in front of fellow players and fans. Frustrated teammates criticize each other, even to the degree of scolding or ridiculing. Up to a certain point, periodic outbursts like these can indeed be motivating. However, when scalding remarks are repeatedly made, akin to bitter husbands and wives who constantly argue, the relationship is on its last legs. For example, at a July 2006 FIVB tournament in Paris, the outspoken Youngs angrily tongue-lashed her partner, Wacholder, in front of a stunned crowd. The ever-intense Youngs broke a cardinal, yet unspoken sports partnership rule, choosing to "diss" her partner in public. The usually reserved Wacholder, visibly upset by these remarks, then uncharacteristically countered with ridicule and anger.

The Domino Effect

This nasty argument, heard around the beach volleyball world, prompted this second-ranked team to disband, triggering a ripple effect throughout the entire unsuspecting ranks. Because the top-rated and secure May-Treanor/Walsh team was untouchable, Youngs and Wacholder began courting the rest. Through a series of overseas calls back to the States, they set the gears in motion. On the receiving end were women who, of course, were eager to compete with either of them. Once these instigators found partners, these two recruited players then abruptly dumped their own teammates. Then, each dumpee had to hurriedly seek another sidekick, thus contributing to the splitting of another duo. This rampaging cycle continued, and when this swirl finally stopped, each of the impacted women landed in the arms of a new companion.

But what about all the months of practicing, training, and goal-setting? All of a sudden, none of that mattered. In specific cases, these new unions were a relief to those who were struggling because they gained new confidence and energy. In other instances, however, these match-ups were casually accepted as a stopgap alliance, lasting just long enough to ride out the season.

Wacholder and Youngs each emerged from this free-for-all with a prized, taller partner. Little did the 6'0" Youngs realize that her choice of the 6'2" Branagh would set off yet another chain reaction

within the AVP months later. Their "Tall-Tall" pairing is now pro-
pelling other duos to follow their lead, challenging the Tall-Short
model. In this new, untested scheme, both players can share all roles
– blocking, spiking, setting, and digging – thereby providing different looks that their opponents must adjust to. They have embraced
this format, successfully dominating at the net and defending in the
back. As Youngs put it, "We're Tall-Tall, but we move very well. We
both play defense and are great at serving."[21]

In 2007, the experiment progressed with tall women's (greater
than 6' tall) and men's (greater than 6'6") teams starting to form.
On the women's side, the aptly coined Big Girl Scramble shook up
the ranks at mid-season. Kicking off this trend, the 6'4" Dianne
DeNecochea left her 5'6" close friend, Barb Fontana, in the dust,
joining with the 6'1" Logan Tom. "I just saw this as an opportunity
to play with a player who is a little bit taller and a little bit more powerful," said the hopeful DeNecochea.[22] Following this lead, the 6'3"
Alicia Polzin paired with the 6'2" Jennifer Snyder, thereby forming
her sixth different partnership in the 2007 season, a number likely
destined for the record books! Several middle-ranked teams got
caught up in the mix, and gave this scheme a try despite these taller
players not being known for their quickness and defense. After a few
weeks, DeNecochea gave up, ended the separation, and reconciled
with the welcoming Fontana. "It just wasn't a good fit," said the re-
gretful DeNecochea. Coincidentally, on the men's side, Fuerbringer
and his 6'6" partner, Sean Scott, also trialed this strategy during
the first half of the 2007 season. But, they struggled with their new
roles – floundering like fish out of water. After several weeks, Fuerbringer returned to reunite with Jennings, and they went on to win
the season-ending Best of the Beach 2007 event.

All in all, the Tall-Tall experiment is still in its infancy. Although
time will tell whether bigger is better, the tide seems to be turning.

Many players believe that this model is the future for Pro Beach Volleyball. They point out that this trend is simply following the lead of other major sports: basketball, football, hockey, and indoor volleyball. But does this model have the staying power to last? Wacholder's partner, the 6'1" Tyra Turner, contended that, "The game is developing into that. Girls that are 6'1" can play defense. They're quick enough and they take a bigger area when they block. And offensively, when they dig a ball, you don't have to set them perfect."[23]

What will become of these "small" players? They still stand a chance, especially those who are young, crafty, and strong – traits needed when attacking against a big blocker. The young 5'3" Chrissie Zartman said, "When you're shorter than almost everyone else, you need to work extra hard."[24] Fortunately, these budding players in their twenties have an edge. On the other hand, height-deprived veterans, those slowed by age and injury, have more difficulty selling themselves to promising taller players – even to those who could benefit from their seasoned wisdom and experience. Therefore, each has two options: settle for another 30-something "old-timer," who is in the same boat, and then struggle to finish in the top twenty at events; or simply retire.

The Real Cost of Divorce

On the AVP tour, winning, and not absence, makes the heart grow fonder. Looking ahead, the partner shuffle will certainly continue if the 2007 season is a barometer. Needless to say, several of the top ten men's and women's teams did not last the entire 2007 campaign. As long as a player believes he can succeed with another, his partnership will dissolve as a new opportunity arises. Among the players, it's "All for One, and One for Me." For better or worse, players have grown to accept the partner-swapping lifestyle.

The real cost of divorce is felt throughout the entire Pro Beach Volleyball community. Due to all this upheaval, the AVP, sponsors, media, and fans are fed up with this whimsical subculture. The AVP is valiantly trying to stabilize the sport, as a foundation for growth. This churn has possibly led some executives to derisively joke about forcing partners to sign a prenuptial, with provisions mandating that players stick it out *at least one* entire season.

That utopian vision alone would merit a standing ovation by all. Sponsors would obviously prefer to support a team so that their brands would get greater exposure. If the partners separate, their investment is out the window. Also, media publications are reluctant to run stories about teams for fear that, by the time an article about a pair goes to print, the two athletes would have already split. It's happened all too often. Finally, the fans, akin to those in other sports, enjoy following a favorite team. In this climate, that's nearly impossible to do. A team cheered on one week may be history the next. Can you imagine your favorite basketball team disbanding, right in the middle of the season, and returning with a whole new lineup? And some of your favorite players are now competing on a team you hated? Would you still be interested? Clearly, in the court of fan opinion, it seldom pays to build any allegiance for these teams.

"Good chemistry is not always easy to come by. When it really matters and starts to show (or disappear) is when you're in a three-game battle and the score is tight. How do you feel when you look over at that person? If there is total trust and you feel relaxed, you've found a winner," said Mason.[25] The problem, beach volleyball players must recognize, is that "total trust and respect" doesn't develop within a fraction of a season.

Eleven

TRICKS OF THE TRADE

"**B**each volleyball was so hard because all the hours training, cold morning workouts, travel, and tournaments. I asked myself how much longer am I going to kill myself for this. Now I'm glad I was able to stick with it," said Rachel Wacholder.[1]

As the only true U.S. professional beach volleyball tour, the AVP is a beacon, of sorts, summoning the athletes to play in the sport they love, to compete among the best in the world. Each year, thousands of eager players pursue their dreams, seeking to earn a spot on the tour. Yet only dozens of players are able to survive this ordeal – physically, mentally, and financially – year after year. Confronting all the off-court challenges is harrowing enough... the restrictive contracts, the sizeable expenses, the low pay. Yet despite this frustrating backdrop, they tackle the court head on, sand traps and all.

Nearly all the athletes who compete in the AVP have played indoor college volleyball. For the top athletes who want to go pro, only two options exist: compete internationally in any number of indoor leagues (since none exist in the U.S.), or play in a domestic beach volleyball tour. Rather than continue competing on an overseas, bone-jarring hardwood floor, many choose to compete at home on a sand court in a sport that is among the safest of all. "My body was always sore from playing indoors and on the beach, it seems like I can play all day," said Albert Hannemann, a 15-year AVP veteran.[2]

Going Outside to Play

As players jump into the footloose beach game, they leave behind a formal, regimented game where team members have an assigned area on the court, perform a role cast in stone, and follow a set of well-rehearsed plays. They enter a brave new world that many assert is more physically and mentally demanding. "You can be a great indoor player and come out here and find little success. But if you put in the time, you can make adjustments. If you can get confidence out here, that is a big help," said Michelle More, a four-time all-conference player at Nevada-Reno.[3]

For starters, on the sand everything is a bit slower: chasing down a ball, getting into the setting position, approaching the net for an attack. To compensate, players must develop "sand legs" – the ability to glide over the sand quickly and lightly. Former indoor players also find that setting, digging and hitting rules are much tougher on the beach. For example, to effectively hand-set the ball, there must be minimal spin. The smaller court requires an adjustment too, especially when serving and spiking so that hit balls do not sail off the court. University of Southern California standout April Ross transitioned to the sport in 2006, a year full of struggles for her. "Everything was much more complex than I ever though it was," said Ross, who has paired with Jennifer Boss to make a run for the Beijing 2008 Olympic Games.[4]

For many, the learning curve can be too overwhelming. Even players, who have ridden a wave of success on national championship squads, quickly drop out, not wanting to start at the bottom in a new sport and work their way up the ladder again. One exception, however, is Brad Keenan, a four-time All-American at Pepperdine University in the 2000s. In just a couple years, he has overcome several challenges on his way to the elite level. "The beach is demanding dude. You can feel like an idiot out there."[5]

A player is indeed exposed – in more ways than one. First, the weather can prove problematic. Pelleting rain causes slippery misplays, gusting wind forces balls to unexpected spots, and even falling snow impacts vision, as occurred in Lake Tahoe, Nevada in September 2006. Second, with only two players covering the whole court, each must be ready on every play to keep the ball alive. This doubles game requires a jack-of-all-trades style because both partners must perform all skills, and any shortcomings are sure to be exploited by an opponent. "On the beach, if you can't do something, you will absolutely be abused for it," said Jeff Nygaard, an Athens 2004 Olympian.[6]

Practice Makes Perfect

To prepare for competition, players frequently hold two-a-day sessions soon after the winter holidays. They split their time between the gym and one of the beaches in southern California, where most players live. From January through March, during this preseason, their painstaking training regimen includes cardio, weights, and Pilates. "The hardest thing for most players is being willing to put in all the work that it takes in the gym," said Dianne DeNecochea.[7]

AVP's Dirty Little Secret

Injuries on the AVP tour are commonplace – part of the beach volleyball landscape. However, what occurred to Jeff Nygaard in 2007 rocked the close-knit volleyball community and caused each player to revisit a taboo topic. Concerned about an unusual sore, he went to a doctor who diagnosed him with an early stage of melanoma cancer, attributed to sun exposure over the years. "I'm scared to death," Nygaard admitted. "It's the worst news I've ever received."[13] Soon afterwards, surgery on his left bicep was performed to remove the cancerous tissue. Despite being cancer-free today, Nygaard wears a shirt on the court and applies more sunscreen lotion. After hearing this news, players suddenly began to talk more openly about this hazard. Their customary views about their bronzed bodies' appeal to sponsors, fans, and marketers were challenged, and many increased their use of protection from the sun. In obvious damage control mode, Leonard Armato callously said, "There are health benefits from being in the sun, but no one should overdo it. We stand for a healthy, active lifestyle. We're not as dangerous as football."[14]

Then it's on to the chilly courts at Manhattan Beach, Hermosa Beach, or Huntington Beach, where the players practice in leggings and long sleeves as protection from the cool ocean breezes. The game's fundamentals are routinely practiced several days a week, until both partners are comfortable that a strong base has been formed. During breaks from these repetitive drills, they polish their strategies by scrimmaging with other teams, a few of whom have traveled from Canada or even China to train with the best.

This formal regimen, far removed from the simple 1970s "play 'til you drop" era, is a reflection of the technological and economic times. Methodical courtside preparation as well as state-of-the-art conditioning and nutritional programs serve as a strong foundation that will carry players through the tiring season. "I put a lot of emphasis on off-season training. My goal is to be prepared to play five matches a day," said Angie Akers.[8] She recognizes that once the jam-packed nationwide tour begins, with tournaments on most all weekends, regrouping teams barely have time to polish their skills let alone maintain their fitness. And Nygaard seconds the motion, "Conditioning is a game dimension that tops the list for making it on the AVP. After a grueling two-day climb to the finals, having that little extra from your preseason conditioning is rewarding not only by giving yourself a greater chance to win, but also because you can walk away in good shape and not crawling in pain."[9]

While players continue training and competing together, their improvement gains are less dramatic and in some cases, imperceptible. Highly-refined skills separate the best from the rest. After hundreds of hours of competition, the game becomes a complex mix of Xs and Os for this finely-tuned machine. A set of a motionless ball, a spike that just nips the end line, or a block that penetrates an extra inch – all can equal an extra point that may decide a game. "It's the little things that count. You need to work endlessly on them," noted the analytical Rogers, aka The Professor, who has been instrumental in teaching his partner, Dalhausser, the finer points of the game. As one example, Dalhausser's repeated setting of the ball at a certain distance from the net has reaped rewards at tournament time, with Rogers' attack game greatly benefiting.

Season after season of competition rewards these athletes with an improved perspective about the game. Many believe the prime age for excelling on the tour is between 28 and 32. By that point, the players are training and playing smarter. It's amazing how players, especially veterans, always end up in the right location on the court. And that's not just pure luck. Over time, the skillful digging

Coaches for Hire

A beach volleyball coach is a luxury that only the elite teams can afford. At a cost well into the tens of thousands of dollars, these coaches, many former AVP players, not only teach players the game, but also serve as sounding boards, and even parental figures for the younger upstarts.

Coaches are indeed an extra set of eyes and ears, and become part of the team. The most well-known coach is Dane Selznick, a USA Volleyball National Coach of the Year, who has led many teams to the victory podium. For instance, while relying on his seasoned experience, he pinpointed all-so-subtle improvements (e.g., striking of a spiked ball, positioning of fingers for a set) to sharpen during practices. Misty May-Treanor and Kerri Walsh are indebted to him for guiding them to their Athens 2004 Olympic Games gold medal victory.

Other coaches certainly love the chance to teach what they have learned. "I have the best ingredients. My job is figure out how to mix them the right way," said former AVP star Liz Masakayan, who has coached several top players.[15] For instance, she is often seen at events charting the plays during matches to share with Elaine Youngs and Nicole Branagh. After discussing the needed adjustments during breaks, the players return to the court with extra ammo and confidence.

And some coaches serve as counselors who need to be in tune with the players' hearts and minds. Mike Dodd imparts not only volleyball knowledge but also fatherly advice. He has successfully mentored the young team of Jake Gibb (youngest of 11 children) and Sean Rosenthal (raised without a father figure), each lacking a minimal foundation of indoor volleyball experience. Since pairing up in 2006, they have learned to lean on him for support and guidance both on and off the court. "I feel like an older brother to Jake and somewhat of a father to Sean," Dodd acknowledged. "I've enjoyed developing these guys as young men."[16] In just a few years, this team has risen to the elite level, even eyeing a 2008 Olympic bid.

of a ball or the strategic spiking to an open spot become second-nature, a "don't think, just act" reflex. For instance, the now-retired Karch Kiraly, a 24-year veteran on the tour, was well recognized for being on autopilot – intuitively knowing how to best dig a ball to the setter, and how to exactly cut a spike. His calculating mind was inherently programmed, and his body was well trained to mechanically respond.

The Game Inside the Game

Can a team rely only on methodical conditioning and structured practicing to get to the top? Only if it wants to "get served" by its opponent. So, each athlete must not only be prepared physically, but also be ready mentally. As the game starts, a player must live in the moment. Volleyball players often speak about competing in the zone – a seemingly invincible aura in which the ball can be clearly seen during each play. With this intense concentration, the players make minimal mistakes and ignore any distractions, thereby improving their play and boosting their confidence. "Once the whistle blows, I'm totally focused. I don't notice the fans or the announcer," said the no-nonsense Elaine Youngs.

For some, this state of mind is difficult to achieve, especially for newcomers still striving to simply master the challenging physical skills. For instance, in his early AVP years, Dalhausser sometimes had difficulty remaining mentally in the game. During a contest, he would often momentarily check out, as if in a trancelike state – a condition players and friends have jokingly coined "Philville."

Even for the experienced, this mystical realm unfortunately comes and goes – sometimes without warning, yet sometimes slowly slipping away along with any momentum. Players resort to all types of techniques to first achieve this inner sense, and second, to maintain it. Kerri Walsh has admittedly had troubles keeping focused during play. As a practitioner of Budokon, an art with meditation and yoga qualities, she often takes a few moments between plays to take deep breaths and refocus. This practice, that translates into "Warrior, Way, Spirit," has "taught me the importance of having strength and balance mentally."[10] Whatever works!

As a rule, beach volleyball players are indeed devious by nature. Case in point, the way some mastermind breakups from their unsuspecting partners. This deception certainly carries over to game time. Any extra point won through mind games can impact the game's outcome. Beach volleyball is as strategic as any other competition where, with each play, the adversary is sized up and challenged.

For starters, players wear "game face" masks as a cover for any frustration or disappointment. Just like poker players, they too hide behind their sunglasses to disguise any furtive glances at open court areas, or even frustration with themselves. Also, just like a wide receiver jukes a cornerback, a beach volleyballer may mix it up by attacking the ball "on-two" rather than setting to his partner. Next, a sly player must key on his opponent too. Sometimes an observant player can read an unsuspecting foe like an open book – with bold print. For instance, a competitor's awkward digging platform may belie a shoulder injury that can be capitalized on by continually serving down the line, just like a tennis player would serve to the backhand of a player whose wrist is taped. In other cases, an opponent's subtle movement that is innocently repeated may be the only opening to seize. For like the chess player who unconsciously plays his pawns in the same way, an inexperienced blocker may stretch his hands too far apart. By detecting this habit, the perceptive attacker can swipe the ball off the blocker's hands and out of bounds for the point. "I have a special talent where I can watch someone play and pick upon what they do well and what they do poorly," said Rogers, well known for dropping short serves just over the net, and out of reach of a tired and struggling player.[11]

Finger Flicking Good

Players need to "finger talk" to each other to prevent opponents from hearing their strategy and to quickly communicate their next moves. Before a serve, or sometimes in the middle of a rally, one teammate will flash a signal behind her back – out of the opponent's view. By using two hands, each representing a side of the net, the partner is motioning how she plans to block. Here's an explanation:

- 1 finger pointed downwards: Player will block the line
- 2 fingers pointed downwards: Player will block the angle (or crosscourt)
- Fist: Player will block the ball, wherever and however it is struck by the attacker
- Open Hand: Player will not block – but may choose to fake going up to the net.

By understanding how her teammate is planning to block, the back-row partner can cover the court left unprotected by the block. This practice has been used for years and is quite effective. But it's been known to backfire – in cases when the opponent's family members see these signals and, in turn, motion the play to them, from afar.

Therefore, each match is a complex battle. Each tournament weekend, teams are constantly fighting off opponents who try to keep them off balance and out of rhythm. And it is increasingly difficult to maintain focus, especially when their bodies are giving out over the course of a drawn-out season. "Beach volleyball is intimidating. It's hard. It's not easy to step out here and challenge the best," said Holly McPeak.[12]

Meanwhile, as these pros do everything they can to prepare for each season, match, and point, the AVP is busily planning its tournaments. Not surprisingly, that task comes with its own set of frustrating and often unusual obstacles.

Twelve

PLANNING MAKES PERFECT?

As Tropical Storm Barry unexpectedly pounded touristy Tampa, AVP officials, players, and fans scurried for cover. Torrential curtains of rain swathed across the AVP's man-made tournament site, spawning newly-formed rivers that streamed past these makeshift sand courts. Matt Gage, the ever-cautious Tournament Director, surveyed the site and reluctantly suspended tournament play, knowing full well that the AVP's best laid plans for this 2007 season event were sinking. Just another weekend in another turbulent season, and another unplanned and unwanted setback for the AVP whose goals of attracting fans and sustaining profits were impacted.

Ever since the AVP's start in 1983, the outdoor tour seasons have been streaky. During the initial years, the player-led organization retained the sport's grassroots vibe due, in part, to its limited finances and its worship of the game. Tournaments in the 1980s were predominantly held in California, as the ever-evolving organization retained the sport's tradition. Courts with weathered wooden poles serving as boundaries, and ungroomed sand pockmarked with hills and valleys distinguished this laidback beach volleyball era from others. Then, during the roller-coaster 1990s, the lively tournament scene reached an annual peak with tens of thousands converging at two dozen well-orchestrated, commercialized weekend parties that stretched across the nation. But, by 1998, the AVP's nosedive into bankruptcy caused these popular events to disintegrate into ghost towns. "The tour used to be kind of dinky," said Leonard Armato.[1]

Therefore, he sought to build up the AVP's tournament image during his tenure in the 2000s. In 2007, approximately half of the 18 outdoor tournaments were held on the west and east coast beaches. There, the warm ocean breezes, sea spray, and soft sand were a throwback to the bygone years. However, to extend its brand and stimulate interest nationwide, the AVP boldly ventured further inland, the last frontier. A ballsy move for sure, because these events were daringly conducted at non-beach locations such as community parks, sports centers, and even parking lots in such landlocked states as Arizona, Kentucky, and Ohio.

Darts Anyone?

Identifying new markets across the nation is difficult for the AVP. For each metropolitan area considered, management assesses such factors as population statistics, local ratings for televised sport shows, indoor volleyball player population, and the hosting of other prominent sports. Also, the AVP must schedule its tournaments within a six-month window, stretching from April to September, thereby allowing for very few "off-weekends."

The elongated and painful scheduling process for outdoor events begins practically a full year ahead of time. Certainly the AVP needs all the time it can get as it evaluates seasonal weather conditions, tournament site availability, and corporate partner preferences. Tough negotiations ensue, with local governments, sponsors, and even television broadcasters each having their own say while understandably wanting their own way... *"Our city's public park is only available in May." "We're not promoting our new product in that market until the summer." "Our TV network's lineup is already full for that weekend."* But lacking the clout of other sports leagues that are held in higher regard, the AVP must often yield to all these demands and constraints.

Here's a sampling of the behind-the-scenes, give-and-take bargaining for the 2007 season:

➤ Tempe, Arizona – City officials demanded that the AVP pay for additional expenses, and reimburse the city for damage to its park due to trucked-in sand for the 2006 event. The AVP balked at these requests not outlined in the agreement. Solution: AVP held the tournament in nearby Glendale instead.[2]

➤ Boulder, Colorado – The city government wanted to host its third straight event. However, the city's available weekends did not mesh with the AVP's. Solution: AVP ended the series.

➤ Any beach, California – The overzealous and overprotective California Coastal Commission (CCC) has persistently been a thorn for the AVP. Its lame policy of ensuring that "the public have access to the beaches for free" butted heads with the AVP's financial goal to charge admission to events in southern California. Therefore, the

AVP threatened to stop holding events in California, even at the most hallowed of all sites, Manhattan Beach, with its decades of steep tradition. Solution: Via public hearings in early 2007, the CCC relinquished and eased its restrictions on admission fees.

The AVP faces this juggling act every year and barely manages to publish its finalized, outdoor season schedule within a few weeks of the season opener. That leaves very little time for all the players, sponsors, media, and fans who need to make travel plans. This belated act is seen by many as evidence of the circus atmosphere of chaos and mismanagement within the executive ranks. In contrast, the stable ATP tennis and PGA golf organizations release their schedules several months before their tours start, fostering credibility and confidence in their tours.

Selling Out

Similar to competitive events in other sports, every AVP tournament is a drain on the bottom line. Gate revenue, approximating a few hundred thousand dollars, covers only a portion of the one million dollars needed to run each event. Therefore, the AVP is always trying to cut its on-site costs. Starting in 2005, the AVP began franchising its tournaments to sports and entertainment marketers that had a strong presence in the selected metropolitan area. Under this promising arrangement, the local promoter signs a contract to not only market the event but also to support the running of it. "We look at the quality of our local promoter and their capability to help us reduce cost and generate local revenue," said Armato.[3] By paying the AVP a license fee, the promoter receives a large percentage of on-site tournament revenue: ticket sales, parking, and concessions. Though the AVP still conducts the tournament, this firm handles such ancillary duties as building the stadium, setting up the courts, and supplying staff for the ticket gate, security, and concessions. Thus, the responsibility for ensuring a great turnout is picked up willingly by the promoter who already has an advertising team and local connections to use its "pull power" to draw people to an event.

For the AVP, what's not to like? Of course, it benefits by not having to devote time and money, sometimes ineffectively, to advertise these events as well as meet with the local jurisdictions for permits, authorizations, and other administrivia. Plus, the risk is transferred to the promoter, who bears the financial burden if an event is poorly attended or if bad weather strikes, for example. However, due to varying unfavorable factors (e.g., unexpected costs, poor weather, low attendance), local promoters used their leverage in 2007 to negotiate a revenue-sharing, instead of a license-fee, arrangement. Buckling under these demands, the AVP shifted to this scheme in 2007 and took a hit, losing $750,000 in income.[4]

In 2007, approximately half of the tournaments were locally promoted, and most all were held at inland locations that required an artificial beach scene with truckloads of sand delivered to form the courts. Some devout beach volleyball purists and old-schoolers still scoff at the AVP for pursuing these man-made locations. They claim it takes away from the sport's allure and its traditional beach vibe. But, the beach can and should be exported to attract fans that may otherwise not be able to attend distant beach contests.

Certain promoters have found success as franchisees. For example, Reach Event Marketing is considered by many to be the frontrunner among the AVP promoters. Leading by example, this Cincinnati firm signed a multi-year contract with the AVP to handle the tournament at a tennis center. Known for its "We Sell Fun" motto, this firm has set the standard for all its peers by specially catering to the players, uniquely reaching out to families, and creatively partnering with sponsors. This company is envisioning even bigger success in upcoming years, thanks to 30,000 fans who attended its 2007 AVP tourney.

Looking ahead, the AVP seeks to steady, if not increase the number of locally promoted tournaments. If a tournament is profitable and enjoys a big fan turnout, like Cincinnati, the AVP will probably come back. Yet, it realizes that some partnerships may financially fizzle. In 2006, for example, a first-time AVP local promoter, Bruno Event Team, held a tournament in the Birmingham (Alabama) Barons minor league baseball park – the same stadium in which NBA-legend-turned-MLB-hopeful Michael Jordan made his 1994 debut. The ballpark was converted into an AVP beach scene by trucking in thousands of tons of sand for the several courts. The question was, could locals be coaxed to attend? At this location in the Deep South, the answer was a resounding "No." Sitting in bleachers to catch the action on the ball field, versus sitting in soft sand courtside on the beach, may have been too much to ask of these new fans. Only a few thousand attended each day, in sharp contrast to the 10,000 fans who packed the stadium to see Jordan compete, albeit at a .202 batting clip. This partnership was temporary, for the AVP did not return for the 2007 season.

All Work and No Play

As these negotiations wrap up just in time for the outdoor season, AVP management is busily working on two fronts: preparing for its own managed tournaments, and coordinating with the local promoters to ensure their plans are on track and that the tournament experience will meet AVP guidelines. While keeping the fan in mind, the AVP decides on the site layout, main stadium seating, size of the tournament field, and ticket pricing (ranging from $10 to $70) for day or evening sessions. To ensure a smooth operation, the planning of a tournament's logistics also takes place well in advance. The tireless Scott Moore, AVP manager of tournament operations, said, "I fly out to sites before the season to check them out. For each new city, I conduct a site survey to determine which is the best layout to use." For instance, an AVP tournament was held in April 2007 at a Dallas site for the first time. Before the season, Moore traveled to the planned tournament location – a barren parking lot area adjacent to the Texas Rangers stadium – and met with the local promoter. While there, he mapped out the tournament layout, akin to a large county fair, while considering the location of the 4,000-seat main stadium, the peripheral seven courts, sponsor row, restrooms, concessions, and areas of pedestrian traffic flow. He reviewed these plans and his expectations with the local promoter who would be responsible for preparing the site.

Once this upfront planning is completed, the optimistic AVP looks ahead to the season and must continually prove itself at each tournament, because its reputation and image are at stake. The players, sponsors, media, and fans all need to be cared for. Regardless of whether the AVP or the local promoter manages the event, the AVP logo is displayed everywhere – a reminder to all of its brand and responsibility.

Before the Pro Beach Volleyball road show comes to town, there's much to be done just before the gates open. First, for a non-beach site, millions of pounds of sand, regularly rented from sand-producing companies, are trucked in. "Transporting the sand, both in and then out of the venue, is always a unique process with cost only being part of the equation," noted Gabby Roe, AVP General Manager of Events and Partnerships.[5] A supplier must be located who can provide #60 Washed Mason sand that is free of debris (e.g., glass, pebbles). Next, a caravan of 20-ton capacity dump trucks makes the trip to the venue. Once the sand is dumped onto the site, front-end loaders and bobcat rakes are used to level, and then till the courts, each requiring 200 tons of sand. In contrast, for tournaments at beach sites, the existing sand is simply leveled and groomed. Rarely is sand trucked in to spread atop the beach sand, which is normally deep enough.

Then, for an AVP tournament where a local promoter has not been contracted, the AVP's lean operations staff of seasonal workers instead handles the set-up duties. After unloading their tractor trailers, the harried crew is directed by Moore to assemble player and referee tents; build the sponsor booths; furnish the luxury VIP sections with its couches, bars, and buffet tables; set up print media and television broadcast areas; and hang oversized AVP banners and signs. The hustle-bustle is everywhere: chugging tractors pulling loaded carts, and speeding golf carts shuttling busy staff. These contractors, on the road for most of the season, are certainly a unique breed. "I have a great bunch of guys who will do anything to get the job done," said Moore. And just as the tournament begins, Moore's jacked crew is finishing its work and looking forward to a slight break, whether it be crashing at the hotel or heading for the nearest bar.

But Even the Best Laid Plans...

With the on-site preparations complete, the AVP is ready for the crowds. The AVP must ensure that the fans are treated well and that they leave as happy campers – ready to spread the word and return to another event. Many of these competitions run without any noticeable hitches, to the relief of the AVP who is always striving to build its reputation and fan base. However, despite the best of plans, problems can, and do, frequently surface. Some are preventable and some are not. Some can be corrected on-site, some cannot. So, each weekend, the dice are rolled and the AVP crosses its fingers for a lucky seven.

Unfortunately, the dice often don't always land in its favor. For example, high expectations for new venues quickly fizzle come tournament weekend. Take the California Expo inland site in Sacramento. On second thought, maybe we shouldn't! What could possibly go wrong on a spring day in California, at a beach-like venue? Both the AVP and the Sacramento Sports Commission local promoter were optimistic about this June 2006 tournament. According to plans, sand was delivered and dumped onto the parking lots for grooming. However, it was too shallow, not a plus for players who favor a deeper cushion. The courts were scattered throughout the complex, causing fans to wander across melting asphalt searching for their favorite teams. This exertion was compounded by the near triple-digit heat. Frustrated fans sought any shade they could find from the searing rays, sometimes merely comforted by the shadow cast by a parking lot sign! Needless to say, very few fans ventured into the main stadium to sit in the metal bleachers, the equivalent of baking on a hot cookie sheet. Among those few thousand who did show up, many complained to AVP staff, who could only politely smile when requests were made for a mister tent, or map-like directions to the courts, restrooms, and concessions. Afterwards, the AVP responded by writing off this debacle and not returning to Sacramento the next year. But what about the fans' suggestions, quite valid for any summer event the AVP holds? These simple, fan-friendly amenities have yet to see the light of day.

The AVP's 2007 season-opener in Miami was another fiasco. With all the popular beaches frequented by thousands each weekend and bordered by restaurants and bars, the AVP's holding of the event at the trendy South Beach would appear be a sure bet. Not! The Miami local promoter, who handles the Miami Heat basketball team, surprisingly chose an undeveloped site far away from the shore and within an unsafe construction zone. And believe it or not, AVP management agreed to this location – anything to get a foothold in this hot market to potentially earn more fans, and better sell its product. However, because the event was poorly advertised, many unsuspecting fans first headed to the shoreline to search for the tournament venue. And with no stadium in sight, many gave up the hunt, while others persisted and eventually found the location – well off the tourist path. Not surprisingly, walk-up traffic, which the AVP often relies on, was nonexistent. Total attendance for the entire weekend was probably at a record low, with only an estimated few hundred grumbling spectators watching the finals. Even the normally reserved and adaptive players were left shaking their heads. "We come to great cities near the beach and play on parking lots. I don't think it is a good idea," said Jason Ring who understandably restrained his remarks.[6]

Although tournament snafus in Miami and Sacramento could have been prevented by better planning, certain problems are simply unavoidable, like the weather. Both the AVP and the players must grapple with these conditions on the fly, for only in rare cases is competition ever stopped. Fortunately, players learn to adapt to varying weather conditions and flexibly adjust their strategies.

> ➤ Sometimes, teams compete in scorching conditions with 100-plus degree temperatures, high humidity, and hot sand that actually blisters the soles. For example, in the 2007 Glendale, Arizona desert event, players were scrambling for any type of protective footwear and requesting that the

courts be frequently hosed down by the crew to cool off the scorching sand. Many joked about the well-worn AVP marketing motto, "Come see the AVP where the action will be hot all day."

➤ During the morning hours at the 2007 Brooklyn tourney, a thick fog rolled in, blanketing the courts. Teams could barely see their opponents across the net. The strategic-minded, yet joking Mike Lambert said, "I was telling everyone to serve a sky ball – no one would see it coming down."[7]

➤ Wind gusts can cause headaches too. This single factor has caused many a team to either tackle the gusts head-on or throw up their hands in surrender. Players generally favor playing into the wind because they can hammer powerful serves and spikes without much fear of the ball landing out of bounds. But if the wind is swirling, as occurred at a 2007 event in Boston, it offers no advantage to either team. As players faced wind bursts exceeding 30 mph, the simple triad strategy of bump, set, and hit aggravated many as bumped balls missed the setter target, and set balls floated either too far away or even over the net. Players were shaking their heads and cursing. "You have to take the right approach mentally, because that's a whole different type of volleyball. It's who plays the best and who stresses out the least," observed Holly McPeak.[8] While the unsuspecting players were focused on lunging for balls that dipped or stretching for balls that climbed, spectators couldn't help but laugh at these valiant attempts.

Sand Hazard

As if Jason Ring didn't have enough on his mind: climbing the competitive ranks, negotiating with the controlling AVP on behalf of the players, working as a carpenter to make ends meet... On a beautiful morning in Seaside Heights, New Jersey, his busy world came to a frightening halt. Although AVP Tournament Director Matt Gage continually insists that these beach courts are both groomed and inspected before each competition, foreign objects like a small piece of driftwood, a broken seashell, or a fractured glass fragment, are sometimes spotted (or felt). Players generally recognize this as a hazard of the job, with occasional injuries simply treated on-site. What worries most players, however, is that a potentially lethal object might not be combed out. The simple sight of a dirty syringe, whether washed up onto the shore as medical waste, or even discarded by drug users, is just plain scary. But stepping on one during a match, as Ring did, was a gut-wrenching experience he would like to forget.

On his way to a win with partner Matt Olson, he landed on a needle, puncturing his foot. Play immediately stopped, as medics and officials scurried to the court. The visibly shaken Ring asked several questions, quite worried about the threat of infection or disease. After the medics treated his foot, he was instructed by Gage to finish the match so that the tournament could remain on schedule. Despite being preoccupied, Ring and Olson won the match. Moments later, Ring was whisked away to a nearby emergency room. In his absence, the rumor mill began to churn. While Ring's court was being re-groomed, players on nearby courts could be seen competing very cautiously. Fortunately, his injury was tended to and he returned to compete later that day. With assurances provided by AVP staff that all courts would be further combed that evening, the players resumed their customary aggressive play the next day. Just another day at the beach office.

> ➤ What upsets players more is the impact of rain on trucked-in sand that does not meet the grade or depth specifications set by the AVP. For example, when pounded by rain, very fine sand can harden. At the Tampa tournament where rain pelleted the site, the shallow, substandard sand base became quite hard packed as a result. Once the storm passed, Gage resumed play and the athletes returned to the now concrete-like courts to warm up. Karch Kiraly, the affable Granddaddy of Beach Volleyball, immediately said, "This is a brutally hard surface to play on. These courts are just like a bowl filled with sand and water, and the sand just packs down."[9] Soon, other players also objected in fear of risking knee or ankle injuries when jumping or diving for balls. Several even threatened not to compete until the problem was resolved and the court softened. In response, Moore's staff quickly used equipment and shovels to dig trenches so that the excess water could flow off the court. Then, fresh sand was carted in and mixed with the existing sand, and the court was tilled to soften it so that play could resume in the already delayed tournament.

No matter the weather or the conditions, the AVP show must go on – ready or not. After several years at the helm, Armato has led the management team in conducting over a hundred indoor and outdoor events. Even with all its trials and errors, the AVP has increased the number of annual tournaments in the 2000s, hopeful that this growth will somehow buoy itself financially.

However, the fans have not jumped on the bandwagon. The small stadiums are often not sold out on Saturdays and Sundays, and new markets quickly become ex-markets. Due to income from sponsors and the gate barely covering the million dollar event price tag, the AVP has little cash available to reinvest, to better market and grow the tour. All the AVP can do is hope that somehow its tournaments will one day catch fire as a blaze of glory, and not as a fizzling sparkler.

Thirteen

THE SHOW MUST GO ON

Whipping the sun-baked crowd into a frenzy at center court, Chris "Geeter" McGee, the unrestrained Master of Ceremonies, launched into another one of his adrenaline-pumping, near-maniacal, nonstop, fact-filled intros of the players who fought their way to the finals. "And here she is, out of Long Beach State, a Three-time NCAA First-Team All-American, Two-Time MVP of the AVP, Reigning World Champion, and 2004 Olympic Gold Medalist… Misty… May…. Treanor……". As the pulsating bass of Ozzie Osborne's "Crazy Train" pumped through the loudspeakers, the jumping crowd was greeted by "I have just one question for this group. Hey Dallas, Are… You… Ready…?"

Instead, maybe he should have asked, "Hey AVP, Are You Ready?" Leonard Armato maintained a low profile in this April 2007 event, the first time the AVP landed in Dallas since 1999, back when the AVP was bankrupt. A week after the "where's the-beach" Miami debacle, all eyes were focused on this tournament, a typical inland event, to see if the AVP could rebound.

The many months of negotiation, planning and preparation between the AVP and this Hicks Sports Marketing Group local promoter were wrapping up just in time for this weekend tournament. Earlier in the week, the eight sandbox courts, consisting of trucked-in sand, had already been groomed. The 4,000-seat main stadium's framework was already erected. And the AVP operations staff, rebounding from its stint in Miami, arrived in Dallas (the second stop on its six-month-long road trip) to support the local promoter.

By Wednesday, the diverse mix of national and local sponsors swarmed into the bustling scene to display their products and set up contests with hopes of reeling in customers within diverse targeted marketing niches. Crocs staff hung up a varied sampling of its unconventional shoes, the Jose Cuervo Tequila DJ toyed with his sound system, the Microsoft Xbox 360 team installed and tested their interactive gaming consoles, and Nautica reps displayed a stately line of high-end "deck" shirts.

Let the Games Begin

Next, the players arrived, some fortunate to have trained and practiced since the Miami season opener. This preparation was much needed, for well over half of the teams were new this season. Therefore, the partners were still getting used to each other's playing styles and personalities during the honeymoon phase, before breakups would begin rifling through the ranks later that year.

As was typical, two classes of players competed: the Qualifiers and the Main Draw-ers. The minor leaguers and the major leaguers, if you will. Every weekend, the "Qualis" hope, despite the tough odds stacked against them, that they can compete with the big dogs. To prove they could hang and bang in Dallas, they had to survive a one-day, do-or-die qualification mini-tournament. Only the top four men's and women's finishers would advance to the Main Draw (MD) show with its all its fanfare, prestige, and prize money – albeit a distant second to events in other big-time sports.

The AVP frugally conducted this one-day trial, a chance for aspiring players to compete within the shadows of the main tournament spotlight. While fostering beach volleyball's grassroots participation traditions, the AVP once again bled money from its reserves by holding this sparsely attended competition. Land use fees, insurance premiums, travel expenses, and wages for staff and referees far exceeded the revenue gained from the nominal registration fee charged to players.

The Odd Life of the Qualis

In Dallas, and at every AVP event, these stardom-seeking wannabes pay their dues in pursuit of fame and money. The Qualis represent a ragtag bunch, from hopeful teenagers raised playing the beach game, to focused college indoor volleyball graduates making the transition, to whimsical AVP old-schoolers. "It takes a commitment…You have to go at it 100 percent and rack up the credit card bills," said Billy Allen, a promising Quali who someday hopes to firmly reside in the "big league."[1]

Just a few days after learning that they earned a spot in this tourney, all the Qualis hurriedly flew into town by late Wednesday night. To save money, many crashed on hotel room floors. Then, wearily waking up by 7 a.m. on Thursday, these 140 lower-ranked athletes stumbled over to the lifeless site to begin what many hoped would be a lengthy, yet fruitful day of competition. Venturing in, they weaved through an unwelcoming maze of tractors and golf carts driven by workers still readying the grounds. Their first stop: a hand-written, oversized sheet of butcher paper listing the single-elimination brackets for the 65 matches, a far cry from the glitzy scoreboards used in the Main Stadium. The Tournament Director, Matt Gage, directed them to their courts, having already checked these to ensure their correct set-up and that referees had been assigned. With ball bags and water bottles in hand (only the MD players get free water), these second-class teams, who might as well have a "Q" branded on their foreheads, located their courts. And while there's a certain purity to this informality, many Qualis believe this "grassroots authenticity concept" has gone too far. Wishing to remain anonymous, one self-labeled hack said, "Unless I am good enough, the AVP could care less."

From this point forward, it's do or die. Lose once and you're toast. They clawed their way through these trenches hoping to climb up the bracket. Compared to the polished MD competitors, their play was rough-edged as they scrambled for errant digs, haphazardly spiked balls, and missed simple serves. Yet, these partners were fiery and animated – emotionally inspiring each other to hang in there and keep fighting, while supported by a few family members, friends, and bored MD players taking a break from their practices. They scrapped for every point, whether straining to make a play, or groveling with the referees. Among the top teams that survived these four rounds of play, the injured Ty Tramblie said, "Going home and not qualifying? There was no other choice. I had to go as hard as I could (because) you spend a lot of money to come out here."[2] Too weary to celebrate, he limped off the court, favoring his severely sprained ankle. These eight pairs gathered up their equipment and returned to their hotel rooms in hopes of getting enough rest for the MD tournament. While still recuperating from their tiring day of play, they took comfort in advancing because each was assured of at least $400 in prize money, earnings well below their expenses.

For the remaining 90 percent of the Qualis who didn't make it, they left Dallas empty-handed, with a range of emotions. Competing in the sport they love, they gave it their best. Heading to the nearest bar to wash down their disappointment, they relived their lost opportunities: *"If only I had…," "If the ref did not call…"* The more optimistic ones, those that were "close but no cigar," like Allen and his partner, AJ Mihalic, reluctantly departed, intent on still pursuing their dream that will require endless time, energy and money. The sympathetic Phil Dalhausser reflected on his fortunately curtailed Qualifier days, "It's not easy. You have to start at the bottom and work your way up. I just got lucky."

Others only competed in the event as an experiment, testing themselves at this professional level of play. Among them was former Dallas Cowboy star Jay Novacek, who was specially invited by the local promoter to drum up interest. In his one and only match, Novacek got smoked, 21-7, 21-6. "You really gain an appreciation for how tough it is to play volleyball at this level. The people who do this for a living are just unbelievable."[3]

The Main Attraction

As the MD tournament officially started on Friday, everyone had high expectations:

➤ AVP – Anticipating a strong turnout to boost its bottom line

➤ Players – Striving to improve their rankings and earn more prize money

➤ Sponsors – Seeking to pitch their products to a new set of customers

➤ TV broadcaster – Counting on exciting action to assure high viewer ratings

➤ Local promoter – Expecting to recoup its expenses

➤ Fans – Hoping to enjoy the competition

When the doors opened, the entire staff was ready for this three-day show, from the bureaucratic AVP bigwigs who greeted the VIPs down to the energetic ball-shagging volunteers who received a free T-shirt and visor in exchange for their shift work. Unlike other tournaments such as those in California, where general admission entrance was gratis, everyone had to buy a ticket to attend this time around. Of course, the AVP and the local promoter could not think of everything, much to the frustration of these arriving fans. Without the benefit of maps, signs, or greeters, they wandered around the site aimlessly, trying to figure out who was playing where and at what time. Although this casualness can be viewed by some as a throwback to the free-spirited beach volleyball era, for most it smacks of AVP disorganization and disrespect. Two traits not welcomed by a 21st century audience who "wants everything now and with a smile."

As the competition began, the men's and women's MD fields of 24 teams, which were seeded based on their most recent tournament finishes, took to the courts. The eight advancing Qualifier teams competed in the first round, many content simply to have landed a spot in the show. And their reward for surviving that grueling Qualifiers event? A pairing against a much higher-ranked team! Due to this match-up, often against some of the top-rated teams in the world, these qualifiers faced a tough road ahead. Because in the MD tournament, the caliber of play is a formidable upgrade – the game is faster, bigger, and more powerful.

The skilled MD incumbents awaited this wary prey with amusement or, perhaps, even with respect. "These teams have nothing to lose," Misty May-Treanor once said of the Qualis, "They can go for it, and if they make a mistake, they make a mistake. They're going to have to hit a lot harder than they normally do. They're going to have to serve a lot harder than they normally do. That's what they have to do to beat us."[4] Given their experience, elite players like May-Treanor, always seem to get the breaks: serves that zip just inside the line and spikes that land just outside the reach of a diving player. Unlike the Qualis, they don't often fall victim to their own errors. Looking back on his Qualifier experience, Jeff Minc, a steady 2007 Main Draw player, said, "You make dumb mistakes, because you're trying too hard, because you think they are a better team."[5]

Lost Souls

Facing these insurmountable odds, these bottom-feeding qualifier teams rarely win their first MD contest, and they continue their plight into the "Contenders" (the polite term for "Losers") bracket. Here, they have to win to keep advancing, by picking up a victory against another likely first-round loser: a fellow Quali or a lowly-seeded MD pair. However, as is customary in many tournaments, all the qualifier pairs in Dallas went the "one-two-barbecue" route, getting skunked after just two matches. They would make a decent play, and the higher-ranked team simply made a better one. Tramblie and cohort Mike Morrison were among the winless, who would be content to simply watch the rest of the tournament, or fly back home to save on further travel expenses. They took it all in stride, hoping to play better in the next tournament. For all these Qualis, it was a rite of passage because with each successful berth into the

MD, they gain more playing time against higher caliber competition, achieve more confidence, and improve their seeding.

Of course, upsets in the early rounds can and do happen. However, when top-seeded teams are quickly knocked out of the tournament in this manner, their exodus sends shock waves throughout the ranks. That's just what happened to the upper-ranked team, Mike Lambert and Stein Metzger. Their opening contest pitted them against a middle-of-the-pack, 17th seed pair, Albert Hannemann and Ed Ratledge. Normally, a match-up like this would be a slam dunk for any top seed. However, in this close three-game series, Lambert and Metzger were out of synch, with numerous misplayed digs causing off-balance sets, forcing, in turn, awkward hits. Hannemann and Ratledge snatched these opportunities and won. "They took advantage and served well. They put us in some bad situations," admitted Metzger.[6] Then, after receiving post-match guidance from their coach, Jeff Alzina, the duo rested for an hour or so. Next up, a 15th-seed MD pair, Brent Doble and Ty Loomis, who also lost their first match in three games, dropping them into this Contenders bracket. Once more, Lambert and Metzger could not shake their lethargy and continued to make misplays. Their rhythm and timing were surprisingly off. After getting spanked in the first game 21-10, they soon quarreled between themselves, argued with their opponents, and even jawed with the heckling fans, who especially riled Metzger. Losing their cool and focus, they also lost the second game. The two left the sand disgusted, consoled by Alzina once more for several minutes. "You really can't have any letdowns. You have to fight through it mentally to get yourself going," said a frustrated Metzger.[7]

While the MD play progressed into the weekend, all teams tried to remain in the undefeated Winners bracket, a safe haven that minimizes the number of matches played. Many of the top teams used the first round or two to get in the bump-set-hit rhythm. "Day One sets the momentum," said Kerri Walsh who, with May-Treanor, swept their first two matches. "We always want a good start and work the kinks out on the first day."[8]

But that's easy for the World Champions to say; they seldom drop into the Contenders ranks. An early round loss in the Winners ranks can haunt a team throughout the rest of the event, especially in a compact two-day men's schedule like the one in Dallas. Even well-conditioned players start to get tired in the later rounds. Spikes zoom out of bounds, sets start to spin, and serves lose their punch. George Roumain, an AVP 2004 Rookie-of-the-Year, felt the burden of a condensed Friday schedule and the sun's searing rays. His partner, John Hyden, reflected, "It's really tough to come through the Losers bracket, especially in these two-day tournaments. There's just not much rest."[9] The hulky 6'6" Roumain, with his linebacker-like build, stands out among all players – far different from his peers' lean, lanky frames. But despite this strength, during his seven years on the tour he has only competed in about 30 percent of the tournaments. He just couldn't seem to get through a season without some form of injury: fractured back vertebrae, sprained ankles, worn-out knees, a broken finger….

During the tiebreaker game of his third match, Roumain's body slowly began to shut down. Big George lumbered all over the court, valiantly struggling to display a fraction of his superb skills that, under normal circumstances, would shine. As his energy reserve hit rock bottom, he fought to remain on his feet. Like a dazed boxer, he wearily tried to keep focused. During each timeout, as sweat poured down his face, he attempted to regain composure. While he was dousing himself with cool water, everyone – Hyden, his opponents, the referees, the fans – wondered what was happening. Returning to the court, Roumain summoned his energy in bursts, momentarily pounding a set or blocking a spike, like a sputtering, out-of-gas car relying on any remaining fumes. As the three-game match neared an end, many more gathered around the court, encouraging him to continue. But by that time, he could barely stand up while shaking off apparent blackout spells to refocus. With each lost point, he collapsed to the ground, then slowly and stubbornly returned to his position on the court in front of now sympathetic referees, puzzled rivals, and concerned fans. When the final whistle blew, he writhed in the sand – physically and mentally exhausted, while being comforted by Hyden. Paramedics soon arrived and transported him to a nearby hospital for observation and much needed rest.

Mind Over Matter

Besides relying on their physical prowess, teams must employ psychological warfare too. All duos proceed into each match with a game plan, whether it be quick-setting, hitting line shots, and/or tooling off the block. But what may be charted on paper may not play out on the court. These plans need to be flexible, with communications critical in making these adjustments. Just like marriages, openness and honesty serve as the foundation. In the heat of the match, teammates give directions, shout out warnings, and instill confidence in each other. Barbra Fontana, is one of the most vocal players on tour, always calling the shots and encouraging her teammate and fellow mom, Dianne DeNecochea. Between points at their Dallas matches, this fourth-seeded pair often paused to regroup, whispering advice to each other ahead of the next play.

In contrast, some teams adopt a full frontal strategy, challenging their opponents head on. Typically the men will try to get under their opponent's skin by provoking them. Arguments often erupt across the net, with a player getting up in the other's face. However, despite only a net separating the teams, hockey-like brawls seldom break out. Opponents recognize that the big mouths are just shooting themselves in the foot. When Lambert and Metzger were both jawing at Doble and Loomis, the pair seemed to enjoy the berating. Because as their rage increased, so did their lead.

Quiet on the Set

Back in the 1980s, trash-talking was an art form on the AVP tour. Loudmouths like Tim Hovland, Randy Stoklos, and Steve Obradovich would heckle anyone and everyone. No one was sacred: players, refs, and fans all felt the brunt of these tirades. Even innocent passersby on the boardwalk were taunted with insults and one-finger salutes. In some ways, these fiery gibes were far more entertaining than even the competition itself. Unlike their old-school predecessors, players today are less animated and more politically correct. Sure they'll argue a point when they believe they're right, or sometimes just to vent. However, they are routinely self-controlled and serious on the court, presumably due to their collegiate upbringing, the sportsmanlike behavior provisions in their contract, and the continual quest for endorsement deals with corporate sponsors. Elite players like Misty May-Treanor, Phil Dalhausser, and Annett Davis are known for exercising restraint on the court, continually keeping their emotions in check while seldom riling anyone.

Another strategic maneuver, the time-honored sport tradition of forcing game delays to gain an upper hand, is not only alive and well in beach volleyball but is quite possibly unmatched by any other sport. Beach volleyball players take full advantage of the sand and sun, two conditions that can't be exploited by other athletes. Besides strategically calling timeouts to ice a server or catch a breather, players are notorious for postponing the action in any number of ways – all under the watchful referee eye. Dax Holdren, an Athens 2004 Olympian, is recognized hands down by his peers as the top staller on tour. When not arguing with referees about a call, he has relied on other stalling tactics, witnessed in all their glory during his Dallas match. For example, after unsuccessfully diving for a ball, he laid in the sand – pondering his error, its origins, and maybe even, for a few moments, the meaning of life! Then, over the next minute or two, he slowly arose and began the elongated process of wiping off sand from his arms and chest, cleaning off his sunglasses, and even swishing the court sand around in a futile attempt to even it out. These strategic actions were inwardly lauded by his teammate, frustratingly endured by his opponents, minimally tolerated by the referees, and amusingly accepted by the fans. All the while, the opposing server waited impatiently for the ref's go-ahead to resume play.

Another tactic, beneficial not only for stalling but also for seizing an upper hand, is arguing with the referees. It's no surprise that players resort to this form of cunning, one that is commonly used by athletes in almost every sport. During the course of a season, players become accustomed to the referees – their personalities, actions, and behavior. "We know what to expect as we head into a match. Some of them call it really tight and others prefer not to get involved," explained Nancy Mason.[10]

Using this knowledge to an advantage, the AVP players are smart and calculating. A player who challenges a referee may have several objectives, depending on how the game is proceeding. Sometimes the motive may simply be to test the waters. By "working" the ref, the player can gauge how the referee's feeling that day and envision the type of rulings he or she will make during the match. In other cases, the player may argue to steer the ref towards changing the call.

Hans Stolfus, aka The Groveler, called out the referees in a tightly contested Dallas game. After a disputable line call by the secondary Down Referee against his team, he charged the First Referee stand

Call It as He Sees It

The AVP relies on several dozen referees each season, many of whom travel with the tour, burdening an already heavily-laden expense budget. Under the direction of Head Referee Steve Owen, the experienced male and female referees keep pace with the players, working as many nine one-hour matches on a busy day. In a courtside discussion during a 2007 Boston event, Owen spoke about the referee's role. "The biggest challenge is to control player emotions, and to be a calming factor." The toughest calls to make, according to Owen, are "setting, ball marks, and touches," all of which involve a keen eye and "call consistency." He emphasized that each referee must also be a great listener and communicator, maintain good rapport with players, and refrain from being defensive or letting his ego get in the way of a correct call.

Each ref walks a fine line. Sure, the fans love it when the players argue. It makes for exciting play. However, the referee must command respect. Ordinarily, after letting the player vent, the ref then explains the call. In an act of sportsmanship, a player may agree to disagree, and walk away shaking his head while muttering his objections. In other cases, the player will challenge the call, becoming more irate with each additional remark. To appease this player, the First Ref may consult with another referee about the decision. However, rarely will a player's complaint cause a judgment to be overturned. Consequently, if a player still angrily rebuts the unchanged call, the referee can threaten a player with a yellow warning card for unsportsmanlike conduct, or even a red penalty card for misconduct. In the end, the court referees have the final say, and Owen seldom needs to intercede.

to challenge the judgment. "He missed the call. You can't let him do that," Stolfus argued. His purpose was to get the call overruled, and he was unrelenting during this three-minute rant, blasting both refs for their indifference. The results of this tirade? The First Ref issued Stolfus a yellow warning card for unsportsmanlike conduct, and then delivered a red point-loss card for excessive misconduct. He and Scott Wong lost the match, yet finished in a respectable seventh place. In his case, "you win some, you lose some."

All these strategies, as slick as they may be, play an important role in Pro Beach Volleyball – a game of momentum. Akin to other sports, this intangible force is difficult to grasp. But once it is commandeered by a team, the results of the match are oftentimes predestined, and the players, the referees, and the fans can definitely sense this change in direction. It's an aura that helps the team stay in cruise control mode. Because a pair needs any edge it can get, especially on the tour where the talent runs deep.

As an example, in one moment a team will be dominating its opponent on the way to a two-game victory and the next moment the tide starts to turn as point after point is lost. In Dallas, the fourth-seeded women's pair, Fontana and DeNecochea, edged the seventh-seeded team of Carrie Dodd and Tatiana Minello in the first game by two points, 23-21. However, after the break, Fontana and DeNecochea fell flat and began second-guessing themselves, unintentionally altering bread-and-butter plays in their next game. Their hitting percentage declined due to such errors as spiking balls out of bounds or into the net. This downturn spiraled into a notable increase in service faults as well. While witnessing their opponents' struggles, Dodd and Minello felt their confidence rise. They began to compete with greater aggressiveness. Spiked balls were more easily played, and their improved setting boosted their strong hitting percentage even higher. The tide turned and they rolled with it, capturing an impressive 21-14 victory to knot the match.

For these two teams, this rubber game was a brand new start, a clean slate. By this time, the players were tiring both mentally and physically, and had already tried various tactics and plays. Fontana and DeNecochea reconvened at their bench (or rather, two chairs and an umbrella) before this shorter, 15-point game. In situations like these, Fontana reflected, "Once we sit down in the box to go into game three, I am trying to figure out the other team's tendencies and what they will carry over."[11] When they retook the court, it was crucial for them to develop a lead early on, to force their opponents into a deep hole that they would have to fight to get out of. Every play was critical and a point swing could prove deadly, because if they fell behind, there would be far less time to adjust and make a comeback. So right from the start, Fontana and DeNecochea grabbed the momentum by attacking with a vengeance. Their forcefulness caught their flatfooted rivals off guard. As their hitting percentage dropped to zero, Dodd and Minello lost all hope in this one-sided, 15-8 rout.

A Bird's Eye View

Tight matches like the one where Fontana and DeNecochea prevailed attracted fans of all ages in Dallas. Amidst these outlying courts, which flanked the bleacher-enclosed main stadium, spectators strolled through this open area deciding which teams to watch. Very few sports can lay claim to this up-close-and-personal vibe, one of Pro Beach Volleyball's strongest drawing cards. In what other sport can world-class athletes be seen from this vantage point? All the skills, strategy, and emotion are on full display. The competition is almost touchable – as the spirited drama unfolds. Every stretched muscle, drip of sweat, and pained grimace is unmistakably evident. Between plays, the strategizing whispers and secretive flashing of hand signals provide a sneak peek about what lies ahead.

The legendary, 46-year-young Karch Kiraly, competing in his 2007 farewell tour, magnetized the spectators in Dallas. Standing shoulder to shoulder several rows deep, the spectators witnessed this master from a vantage point just a few steps away from the court's perimeter. Fans favored this setting, and embraced this grassroots-era flashback to the late 1970s when Kiraly competed in front of similar crowds as he began his stellar career. Benefiting from this closeup view, they were drawn even closer to the teamwork between Kiraly and partner Kevin Wong (Scott's older brother). Before each serve, the two encouraged each other, and muttered strategies out of their opponent's earshot. As play resumed, quick commands were barked by Wong: "Line!"… "Angle"… to alert Kiraly where to hit the ball.

From this viewpoint, the riveted fans can see how players interact and understand what makes them tick. Beach volleyball fans are a special breed. Many have a strong passion, dedication, and appreciation for the game. They cheer the great plays, moan at the mistakes, and applaud both sides at the end. The Dallas players were indeed boosted by the fans who cheered them on. After each MD match, fans huddled around the players' bench area and patiently awaited the chance to meet the competitors. They know that these unpretentious pros prefer to hang out afterwards, unlike other sports figures who are whisked away in limos with hardly a wave to the crowd. These fan-friendly athletes humbly welcomed all requests for autographs and pictures from fans who shared the same love for the game. "It is a tangible, palpable connect that anybody who comes to a tournament senses on one level or another," said

Jeff Nygaard.[12] By today's standards, these players are at the top of the sports role model chart. For example, in Dallas, the popular pair of Rachel Wacholder and Tyra Turner was extremely approachable and graciously chatted with their followers.

As each match ended, the Dallas tournament proceeded like clockwork per an adaptable schedule arranged by the ever-busy Gage. Match results were called in to him via walkie-talkie by AVP interns and volunteers. He then manually recorded these wins and losses on the two-sided "main board," an approximate 10' long by 6' high oversized placard. This communal gathering point (presumably an AVP cost-savings measure), attracted fans and players alike. The enormous and antiquated board, that captured all the men's and women's Winners and Contenders bracket results, was overwhelming at first for newbie fans. However, as they better understood how the board was used to chart the event's progress, they soon taught others how to interpret the standings, a relief to the hoarse and tired Gage.

With visions of rest and nutrition, the athletes ambled to the Player's Tent, often stopping to chat, pose for pictures, or sign autographs. Then, once within this oasis, the players lounged on sofas, received massages and physical therapy, and helped themselves to a buffet spread including such healthy foods as pasta, chicken, bagels, and fruit. Despite this variety, some players were simply content with making a peanut butter and jelly sandwich. In many ways, they're just Average Joes, like the fans who came to watch them.

While players chilled between matches, spectators trekked through the Dallas tournament site checking out the carnival scene and each other. Whiffs of body oils and barbecue grills filled the air, drawing everyone further into the bustling midway – complete with concessions, of course. Here spectators, having already shelled out between $20 and $40 to attend this all-day session, were encouraged to spend whatever remained on AVP swag.

Along this stretch, the AVP's highly valued supporters set up shop along Sponsor Row. Tents lined each side of this passageway where energetic corporate reps enticed fans to try out such popular products as Microsoft Xbox 360 games, Herbalife energy drinks, and Schick disposable razors (all of whom would not return for the 2008 season). Meandering further through this maze of swimsuit-clad fans showing off their bods, these wanderers unexpectedly stumbled across sponsored players who, as required by their contracts, were holding informal autograph sessions. Suzanne Stonebarger and Michelle More were among the AVP's chosen few to have landed endorsement deals, and were willingly signing anything at their sponsor's table. Strutting onwards, the skilled and not so skilled were tempted by lame games of chance. Wilson Sporting Goods' "guess the number of volleyballs," Barefoot Wines' "serve the volleyball in the bucket," and Sour Punch Straw's "ring the bell with the sledgehammer" helped pass the time, as best they could. Next, with bags full of sponsor freebies and prizes, many checked out the cool Jose Cuervo Tequila tent with its cozy lounge chairs, big screen TVs, and blaring music. The roving DJ enticed everyone to the bikini contest where Cuervo dancers gyrated on a stage to pulsing hip hop. Taking the bait, gawking and hooting males soon rushed to this show for a closer view, as women and children on the periphery exchanged questionable glances. Flanking this commercial zone were oversized inflatables: an official Wilson AVP ball (emblazoned with Armato's signature) and a green Gatorade bottle, both of which were tethered in place due to the strong winds. The last thing the AVP needed was for these treasured sponsor symbols to become dislodged and start rolling around.

The partnering broadcaster, Fox Sports Network (FSN), also commanded the AVP's full respect. Relying on its leverage achieved through its slanted contract with the AVP, it dictated the schedule for the regionally televised men's and women's finals – held on Saturday and Sunday, respectively. Therefore, on the men's side, 45 Main Draw contests, that spanned several rounds of play, were crammed into a 32-hour period. To survive this grueling schedule, teams reaching the semifinals had to rely on their strength and endurance, attained via extensive training and conditioning. For instance, Ryan Mariano and Larry Witt tumbled into the Contenders bracket after losing their third match on Friday. With play resuming on Saturday morning, they faced an uphill battle. Yet they won their next three matches, knocking out one pair after another, leading up to the "Crossover" semifinal round where the two undefeated Winners and the two single-loss Contenders teams competed. Lose here and you're history. Mariano and Witt, already at a disadvantage after fighting through six matches, were greeted by the unbeaten and well-rested favorites, Todd Rogers and Dalhausser, who had skated through the Winners bracket in just three matches. But the underdogs hung tough, during this warm and windy day, taking the leaders to three games before settling for a well-deserved third place.

As the men's competition was nearing an end on Saturday, the women were progressing through their three-day schedule, with most matches refined to the Contenders bracket. This format allowed Winners bracket teams to rest for most of the day. When not playing, these undefeated pairs relaxed in the Hilton Hotels sponsor's nearby property or remained at the site to check out the competition. In any case, throughout the day all 24 teams competed, realizing that only six of them would advance to Sunday's action. Ashley Ivy, a rising star on the tour, finished her day in the

13th spot that earned her a mere $850. "Making the jump to the top eight teams is a huge undertaking. And all the teams that you see on Sunday (semifinals) – we're right in the matches against them," she said.[13]

Welcome to the Show

Fast forward to the Finals events, pitting Rogers/Dalhausser against Jake Gibb/Sean Rosenthal, and then May-Treanor/Walsh versus Elaine Youngs/Nicole Branagh, one of the few Tall-Tall teams on the women's tour. These championship contests were held in the 4,000-seat Main Stadium, the heart of the AVP tournament. Although preliminary matches were earlier played there in front of sparse crowds, the AVP finally held its official "open house" and showcased itself to all – while relying on its partners' support. FSN, after hours of set up and testing, had its cameramen and commentators poised for the start. The nervous local promoter ensured that its own VIPs were comfortably seated. The national sponsors checked that their banners were firmly affixed and in view of the TV cameras that would pan the stadium during timeouts. For the fortunate subset of firms whose sponsored athletes made the finals, they proudly awaited their bonus, the bodily display of corporate logos that would be shown on TV. Last, the anxious AVP staff – ranging from the summer interns handing out noisemakers, to the operational staff testing the Jumbotron screen one last time, to the commanding AVP management overseeing the activity from the main stage – hoped for another successful event. Show time!

Everyone streamed into the stadium: excited preteens with their curious parents in tow, throngs of teenage girls with signs, 30-somethings sipping icy Cuervo drinks, and the diehard volleyballers wearing well-worn visors. Once inside, they were greeted by this intoxicating fanfare, awash with colorful banners that surrounded the electrified main court. Welcoming these fans were the resounding lyrics from the old-school, classical rock legends Emerson, Lake, and Palmer, blasting through the loudspeakers...

Welcome back my friends to the show that never ends
We're so glad you could attend
Come inside! Come inside!
The show's about to start
Guaranteed to blow your head apart...[14]

While watching these elite players warm up on center court, the primped fans, some wearing bikinis and boardshorts, were eager to strut their stuff too, undulating in time to bass-heavy hip hop and rock music. Roving cameramen captured this raw energy and projected it back to the crowd on the gigantic TV screen. The display of sunbaked, hot bods bouncing to "This Is Why I'm Hot" by M.I.M.S. and smacking their thundersticks together in unison, stoked the crowd even more. The lovefest was already underway, well before the first whistle.

Following Geeter's rapid-fire introduction of the finalists, all four players were amped as adrenaline chills coursed through their bodies. They fed off this energy, while relying on their deep reserves of strength, conditioning, and experience that led them to this pinnacle. Competing in front of a packed house against the best in the world was all they had ever dreamed about.

With game strategies rushing through their minds, each team hustled to the net to greet each other. They then seized their starting spots on the court while the four referees manned their posts. With pulsating techno music driving the deafening crescendo of thunderstick pounding, the overcrowded scorekeeper's table could only motion its readiness to the First Referee. He promptly issued a sharp blast from his whistle and extended his arm upward, and then across his body to signal the first serve. As the crowd quieted and the TV camera slowly panned to the server, all attention was now focused on the action.

As both the men's and women's championship matches progressed, initial player nervousness – evidenced by off-target sets, missed spikes, and long serves – soon subsided. The teams soon fell into a groove, resting on a cadence of well-practiced plays. Yet, they were always wary about this rhythm being disrupted by their cagey opponent, intent on gaining an edge.

From the main stage overlooking the court, the irrepressible Geeter stoked the players by giving them props for jump serves that bombed the corner, sweet hand sets that were nectar, and hard-driven heaters that smoked a line. Further, he constantly engaged the crowd. Whether leading a stadium-wide wave cheer, comically providing the play-by-play for a fan contest during timeouts, or playfully teasing couples caught by the "kiss-cam," he engendered even greater rapport. "I consider a tournament successful if an audience member can walk away from the court and say, 'Hey, that was fun!'" [15]

Each game played out as a series of mini struggles. Heightened by crafty serves, acrobatic digs, and precise setting, battles were typically fought at the net. Here each match was waged in mini one-on-one contests, with each player trying to strategically outguess and powerfully outplay the other. For example, Walsh would forcefully swing or cagily cut, trying to drill the ball past the outstretched, suppressive Branagh block to an indefensible spot in the sand. Each point became a small victory, a steppingstone to winning the match.

In Dallas, the contests ended with the favorites and Beijing 2008 Olympic hopefuls, May-Treanor/Walsh and Rogers/Dalhausser, sweeping their two-game matches by near-identical scores. "You do get people gunning for us. You get used to it, and come to expect the best from every team you play," said Dalhausser.[16] In front of the cheering crowds, each team was awarded a modest $20,000 check by the AVP. As they posed for pictures, each player ensured that their sponsors' logos were clearly visible for the fans and TV cameras: the Wilson visor, the Nautica headband, the Hilton Hotels tattoo.... And per tradition, each champion capped off the victory with the shaking and then popping of champagne bottles – spraying TV employees, sponsor staffers, AVP executives, and fans courtside. Reflecting on hard-fought victories like these, May-Treanor said, "Kerri and I work very hard. For us to stay at the top is very difficult because teams are getting better."[17]

By various first-hand accounts, the Dallas tournament was a success – according to the thrilled fans enjoying the beach party, the optimistic sponsors and local promoter welcoming the spotlight, the TV network that featured this event in its lineup, and the AVP fast-talking executives who congratulated each other. "We tried to make it more engaging, have a lot of interactivity. I think fans enjoy the engaging feel. We take some of the world's best athletes and wrap it around the beach lifestyle," reflected Armato.[18]

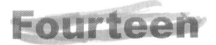

A LINE IN THE SAND

Beach Volleyball captures the world's attention every four years, as one of the most popular sports in the Summer Olympic Games, The fast-action, dance-party, and sexually-charged event attracts hundreds of thousands of spectators and hundreds of millions of TV viewers. With gold medal victories at each of the last three Summer Olympic Games, the U.S. has prevailed on this international stage. The incredible success of the two women's medalist teams at the Athens 2004 Olympics took the world by sandstorm. As Kerri Walsh proclaimed after she and Misty May-Treanor captured the gold in 2004, "The sport is growing and no one's gonna stop it."[1]

No one is going to stop it intentionally, for sure. However, despite this Olympic glory, Pro Beach Volleyball still languishes amidst the American sports landscape. To be sure, the sport momentarily catches the public eye via the Olympic windfall of excitement and intrigue. Immediately after each Olympic Games, players of all ages descend on freshly created courts in neighborhood parks, or rush to the beach to give the sport a shot. Within certain grassroots pockets of the country, newly formed beach volleyball clubs have organized leagues to promote participation. In recent years, the USA Volleyball (USAV) organization, emerging from its restructuring that was triggered by the AVP's Article VIII filing, has ratcheted up its involvement in beach volleyball by holding youth clinics, conducting "open" tournaments to identify promising junior players to foster in its pipeline training program, and grooming elite-level athletes to succeed internationally.

At the Pro Beach Volleyball level, the AVP has tapped into this Olympic momentum to improve its own popularity and profitability. For each of the three Summer Olympics where beach volleyball was contested, the ever-optimistic AVP has timed its marketing campaigns and publicity programs accordingly. And every time it has knocked on the American sports mainstream door, hoping to be embraced by the masses.

However, every four years, the door has opened ever so slightly, just long enough for the AVP athletes who won Olympic medals to enjoy the spotlight and give some props to the AVP through appearances and interviews. But the welcoming is always short-lived. After the Olympic Games' afterglow faded, the sobering AVP has had to retreat and reorganize. For example, subsequent to the Sydney 2000 Olympics, the bankrupt AVP needed a lifeguard to rescue it from ruin. "Without Leonard Armato's intervention, the sport virtually would have died out," said Sinjin Smith, a 1996 Olympian.[2] Then, after the Athens 2004 Olympics, the AVP went public with its company to obtain much needed capital to fund its operations and growth plans.

To Armato's credit, since his takeover in 2001 the sport has thrived in many ways. The improved standard of play, the heightened commercial interest by the media and sponsoring corporations, and the increased fan base are all indications that the sport has progressed. However, the AVP has faced several obstacles in its constant fight to financially survive during each Olympic quadrennial period.

Kinks in the Success Chain

In theory, a chain of marketing milestones, when successfully achieved, should serve as the ongoing guide and the needed sustenance for any sports property. For example, the greater the publicity, the greater the fans, the greater the sport's popularity, the greater the TV coverage and ratings, the greater the revenue negotiated from sponsors, then the greater income the sports organization should have to reinvest for the good of the sport and the players. But in the case of the AVP, not so great! Within its own chain, these links often weaken and the AVP finds itself scrambling to fix them.

There are two major causes for these weak links. First, the AVP's tarnished history still haunts it to this day. The previous mistreatment of sponsor, television, and promoter partners has been difficult to overcome. The AVP is still considered damaged goods, receiving little respect from corporations. By struggling to land even small-scale, short-term deals with prudent sponsors, by relinquishing its rights to broadcast revenue from overbearing networks, and by selling itself out to local promoters, the AVP has missed out on lucrative revenue opportunities that come easy for well-established sports. Second, as the only professional beach volleyball organization in the United States, this monopoly has become complacent, not overly focused on efficiency or innovation. Since 2001, the AVP has been managed by "seasoned" middle-aged males with minimal beach volleyball knowledge. Management has been slow in taking risks and keeping up with the times. For instance, only recently has the AVP ventured beyond the beach by conducting more tournaments inland and indoors, a strategy appealing to corporate sponsors and television networks that favor a larger footprint across the nation.

Right from the start of this chain, the AVP has battled with the publicity link that sets the foundation for this sequence of favorable events. The AVP has an image problem, pure and simple. Management has not effectively marketed the tour on a national level, relying primarily on magazine ads and its website instead. The almighty fan, whether a tournament spectator, a TV viewer, or a website visitor, is worshipped within the sports entertainment world and must be lured to the sport. The AVP has shortsightedly identified its primary audience as 18 to 34 year olds. But, for many within this coveted demographic, the advertised term "AVP" is more likely to conjure up images from the "Alien Vs. Predator" movie than of Pro Beach Volleyball!

Due to this ineffective publicity effort, it's no surprise that the AVP has resorted to smoke and mirrors to sell itself. Specifically, the AVP still claims that it draws one million spectators annually to its outdoor tournaments, and that it is the fastest growing sport. These hyped promotional pitches are unfortunately often ignored by the next link, the TV networks that strive to estimate viewership. The AVP, consistently plagued by low ratings for its tournament broadcasts, has had neither the luxury nor the leverage to negotiate a deal with one prominent network, as other sports routinely do. Instead, the AVP has painstakingly had to manage a hodgepodge of broadcast outlets, to gain as much airtime as possible each outdoor season, in hopes that viewers know when to tune in to which channel each weekend. Given plans to improve its visibility during the 2008 Olympic year, the AVP hired an advertising firm, Creative Artists Agency (CAA) in December 2007. Despite never having represented a sports league, it has been tasked with seeking viable broadcast opportunities.

Of course, low numbers of TV viewers and tournament spectators have caused many sponsors to question the value of their funding – another damaged link in this chain. To be sure, a few major corporations like Crocs, Wilson, and Jose Cuervo Tequila have admirably invested in the AVP for the long-term. However, during the 2000s, numerous corporations, from the startups to the blue-chips, have come and gone through a revolving door. Initially attracted by the "sun, fun, & buns" image and the pompous AVP hype, many got caught up in the lifestyle and vibe, and gave the tour a shot for a year or two. But, once the honeymoon ended, and disappointment, disagreement or even disgust swept in, they departed to seek better opportunities, presumably in other sports leagues. This turnover has continually saddled an already strapped AVP management team that must negotiate, plan, and coordinate with dozens of national and regional sponsors, new and old, each season.

Sponsor funding, as unsteady as it is, represents 85 percent of the AVP's annual income. However, in recent years, this revenue has barely covered the weighty tournament costs, let alone the excessive administrative expenses. Needless to say, the AVP has not reported a profit since its rebirth in 2001. Risk-taking shareholders, both corporate and individual, are furious as they watch their stock investments plummet.

Sadly, each year, there is insufficient cash remaining for the AVP to reinvest in itself, and in the players who clearly are a pivotal link in the chain. These 200 contracted players indeed carry the tour. The AVP relies on these athletes, but its support is clearly suspect.

Its stranglehold grip has choked the players' livelihoods. These "in-dependent contractors," striving to make a living in a game they love, have been held hostage by a contract that limits prize money, restricts corporate sponsorships, and usurps licensing rights. Due to these unfavorable conditions, most all players frequently change partners with goals of earning more money and landing sponsor deals. In turn, these roster shake-ups have haunted the AVP be-cause the inherent team nature of the sport has all but vanished, causing frustration among fans who enjoy following teams.

Furthermore, the high-and-mighty AVP has done little to market its contracted players, especially since it owns their likenesses that it reaps revenue from. The AVP has often contended that it en-courages sponsors to contract with players for endorsement deals, but very few companies have included these athletes in their ad campaigns. In general, player audience appeal is paramount for a sport's popularity. However, unlike other sports whose top athletes are well known, Pro Beach Volleyball players are hardly household names, with the possible exception of May-Treanor and Walsh.

At a Crossroads in 2008

As another Olympic year, 2008 is critical for the AVP. Only a few professional sports, like basketball and tennis, are lucky enough to benefit from boon years like these, where their sport is uniquely showcased for millions in this same world spotlight. For those that do seize this bonanza of attention, their league management often begins planning several months beforehand, and establishes a bud-get sufficient for cranking up promotions, pursuing greater public-ity via the media, and attracting more fans who are newly tuning in to the sport. Investments like these have the potential for long-term payoffs. Therefore, the AVP should similarly be seeking to exploit this advantage.

But is the AVP poised for this challenge during this make-or-break year? Not even close. A busy 2007 season was devoted to operating the 18-stop tour, preparing for the inaugural indoor Hot Winter Nights Tour, and grappling with stockholders over the ill-fated buyout proposal. And even if time was available for this up-front planning into early 2008, there was minimal cash available. With a reported $4 million loss in 2007, the AVP had limited funds to support any plans for publicity and growth.

Of course, the AVP continued to project optimism at every turn. "Looking forward, we remain focused on moving onward and up-ward, growing our business through exciting new initiatives, new strategic relationships, and continuing to explore a flood of other expansion opportunities," as the AVP stated in a publicly filed financial statement commandeered for schmoozing purposes.[3] However, several AVP executives and Board members, including the Chief Growth Officer and other long-time cronies, did not rally behind Armato, likely tiring of this operationally and financially jarring roller-coaster ride. These eight top executives and Board members bailed in early 2008, taking with them all their knowledge and ex-perience, and leaving Armato holding the near-empty money bag. And some of their departures came with a price tag, in the form of expensive golden parachute severance packages.

Several coveted sponsors also pulled out in the off-season despite the prospect of selling their products to a greater base of fans during this Olympic year. This exodus may trigger the departure of several other prominent sponsors like Bud Light, Jose Cuervo Tequila, and McDonald's, whose contracts are expiring in 2008. To partially fill this void, AVP management quickly sought more sponsors, signing up such lightweights as PNY, Affinity Real Water, and American

Laser Centers. However, for the AVP to end its string of annual financial losses, lucrative deals with new, prominent sponsors will need to be negotiated.

Likewise, the support from loyal stand-bys, that the AVP has routinely counted on, has suspiciously fallen off. Despite the popularity of beach volleyball telecasts during the Olympic years, NBC agreed to broadcast just four AVP events in 2008, and Fox Sports Network contracted only to regionally televise events as tape delays, often weeks afterwards. Clearly the CAA advertising firm was not meeting AVP expectations. The coupled link is deteriorating between sponsors who require TV time to sell their products, and the networks that require commercial time slots be filled with sponsor ads. As such, it will be difficult for the weakening AVP to soon restore this union.

Even by the first quarter in 2008, the AVP was already facing a significant and unexpected hit to its bottom line. With its budget reduced, AVP management (or whatever was left of it) had to cut its expenses by scaling back its season-opening Media Day event, decreasing its advertising, curbing its 25th anniversary celebration, and compacting the scope of several tournaments by cutting out the preliminary Qualifier round and limiting the Main Draw field.

All these cutbacks come with a price. Frustrated fans are the AVP's top concern and justly so. Right from the outset of the 2008 season, beach volleyball fans were angered by the much delayed announcement of the tournament schedule and a streamlined website that, due to cost-cutting reasons, no longer provided the fan-favored, streaming videos of live tournament action. So is there anything the AVP could do to ensure the fans are treated well on-site and that they leave as happy campers, excited to spread the word and return to another event? Clearly the expensive, high-tech use of "visorcams" to capture the closeup action on the Jumbotron screen is out of the question!

However, to encourage greater attendance for the events it manages, the AVP should consider only charging admission for its main stadium seating. The lost gate revenue would be favorably offset by increased concession sales and improved visibility of sponsor products. Plus, simple amenities like handing out a program, adding more chairs at the satellite courts and the food stands, and even setting up a water misting tent for fans to cool off during hot days would be welcomed.

Also, the AVP should provide a diversion for the fans to participate in, as a break from watching the matches. Sure there are sponsor contests and an extra court is used for pickup games and clinics. However, senior management should step into the 21st century to further connect with fans not only in its treasured demographic base, but within the youth ranks. By using its extreme sports label to its advantage, the AVP could easily attract a new set of followers.

How? The AVP could introduce some family-friendly activities patterned after the interactive and entertaining Dew Action Sports Tour that features skateboard and BMX action with a backdrop of live music. For example, the AVP should include, as a sidelight, edgy demonstration sports (on the fringe of beach volleyball) such as beach tennis, soccer volleyball, or even "Bossaball," a sport competed on a court of inflatable trampolines. Then, after a brief lesson, the fans could play on the courts that are emblazoned with sponsor logos. These exciting offshoot sports, relatively inexpensive to set up, would further distinguish the AVP and create a buzz in the sports entertainment world.

Value-added enhancements like these are definitely a plus. However, the AVP must recognize that it is the competition that reels fans in. The unique closeness at events between players and spectators fosters a sense of community and affinity, a distinguishing drawing card in a crowded sports market.

This camaraderie is in jeopardy, because of the AVP's oppressive control over the players. The AVP must indeed loosen its reins on these athletes, the last link in the chain of success. The restraining contract terms have sanitized the sport and indirectly curbed its popularity. Ever-cautious players, eager to earn a living, have become workmanlike in their approach to the game. Unfortunately, this seriousness does not translate well to the beach vibe atmosphere and runs counter to the grassroots, fun-loving lifestyle that the AVP promotes.

Fortunately, the players hold more power over the reborn AVP than ever before. The upstart Professional Beach Volleyball Association collective is challenging management's proposed contract, effective in 2009. As the players, ranging from the lower- to the higher-ranked, fight for improved rights and greater financial benefits, they do so not only for themselves but also for the newcomers the AVP will rely on. For these upstarts seeking stardom, a better breeding ground is needed. The AVP's inadequate *AVPNext* grassroots program and the problematic qualification system, now partially funded by tapping into the Main Draw players' payouts, can no longer be relied upon to ready these athletes. The USAV, with the help of its regions, must continue to support a newly emerging, grassroots national system to cultivate teenage and adult talent. Also, for those AVP elite athletes contending for Olympic glory, the USAV must cover travel, coaching and training expenses, as afforded to the indoor players, for the Federation Internationale de Volleyball (FIVB) events. However, with greater backing and higher prize money payouts, the elite players may indeed opt to compete strictly overseas.

To thwart a potential migration of its top players, the AVP must utilize the CAA firm to also market these athletes, shifting this responsibility away from its ineffectual, in-house marketing staff. The former sports agent Armato clearly understands how the power of publicity can boost an athlete's recognition, and in turn, financial livelihood. In this win-win situation, both the AVP and the players would capitalize from increased exposure. The AVP would certainly savor this enhanced public awareness, and the players would benefit, at the minimum, by being featured in a newspaper, magazine, or even on an ESPN show. Given the 200-player population, there are ample opportunities for great stories to be told about the men and women players, the latter appealing to both male followers and to a growing female fan base who consider these players as role models.

In many ways the fate of Pro Beach Volleyball may ultimately lie in the hands of the women. Ever since Armato opened the doors to them in 2001, the AVP has clearly profited from the attention the women have garnered, and in many cases has passively gone along for the ride. May-Treanor and Walsh have embraced their leadership role. "The sport got a major lift in mainstream interest from our performance in 2004. We need to take care of business again," said the confident Walsh.[4]

Recently, however, both women have openly discussed leaving the tour to start a family soon after the 2008 season, hopefully taking their Beijing Olympic gold medals into the delivery room for good luck. Moreover, Armato's wife, Holly McPeak, who has collaborated with him on many a decision, has stated that 2008 will be her farewell season. While no one in the sport would dare to acknowledge it, the foundation of beach volleyball may be shaking.

A Final Rally?

So where does the AVP and the sport of Pro Beach Volleyball go from here? During this Olympic year, the AVP should be fully focused on its tour and promoting itself as well as its players who will be competing in the Beijing 2008 Olympic Games. However, this time around, there has been no knocking on the sports mainstream door. Therefore, without any welcoming acceptance, there will be little momentum to carry into the next four-year Olympiad.

The late 2000s are eerily reminiscent of the late 1990s when the struggling AVP also suffered financial losses, sustained management turnover, endured sponsor desertions, and stomached dismal TV coverage. Due to an unsteady financial footing and a gloomy 2008 outlook, the depleted management team has been forced to retrench, and even reorganize by overhauling its Board of Directors, prompted by a challenge from two prominent investors. And it appears that the AVP is now surrendering and going soft – too tired of playing hardball with sponsors, networks, local promoters, the USAV, and the players. Therefore, the AVP's visions of achieving recognition and progressing up the sports entertainment ladder have faded.

As he considers his future, Armato faces a very difficult "stay or go" decision, one that may be eased by his recently crafted severance package. And if history is any indication, the AVP may require a new savior to rescue the tour and potentially conduct a sweeping makeover. If one isn't found, it may turn out that when May-Treanor and Walsh step away from the tour, the entire sport may also venture into the sunset. Pro Beach Volleyball will then no longer be led by a king and his court, but by a pair of queens.

Appendices

A - HISTORY OF BEACH VOLLEYBALL

B - BEACH VOLLEYBALL TERMS

APPENDIX A
HISTORY OF BEACH VOLLEYBALL – UNITED STATES

1895	William G. Morgan, an instructor at the Young Men's Christian Association in Holyoke, MA decided to blend elements of basketball, baseball, tennis, and handball to create the game of Volleyball. He used a tennis net and raised it to 6'6".
1920s	Most believe the sport was born in Santa Monica, California where the first volleyball courts were set up on the beach, and families played six-on-six.
1930s	Doubles beach volleyball was initially played in Santa Monica.
1947	The first official two-man beach volleyball tournament was held at Will Rogers State Beach, California.
1948	The first tournament to offer a prize was conducted in Los Angeles, California where a case of Pepsi is awarded.
1950s	The inaugural tournament circuit was organized by the California Parks & Recreation Department on five beaches in California: Santa Barbara, Will Rogers State Beach, Sorrento Beach, Laguna Beach, and San Diego. Beauty Contests were added to the tournament program.

1960	The first Manhattan Beach Open was held.
1965	The California Beach Volleyball Association (CBVA) was founded, and rules officially established.
1974	Winston Cigarettes became the first commercial company to sponsor a tournament that offered $1,500 in prize money in San Diego.
1976	Events Concepts Incorporated (ECI) was formed to promote and expand the beach tour.
1978	Jose Cuervo Tequila became the sport's first major sponsor.
1980	The first sponsored tour in the U.S. was organized with seven events offering $52,000 in prize money.
1983	On July 21, the Association of Volleyball Professionals (AVP) was established to protect players' interests and to preserve the integrity of beach volleyball.
1984	AVP players held a strike at ECI's World Championships in Redondo Beach, California. And the AVP began conducting its own events.
1986	An AVP tournament was aired for the first time on network television on ABC's Wide World of Sports. The Women's Professional Volleyball Association (WPVA) was created to organize women's pro beach volleyball events that had previously been played as amateur games or as a sidelight to the men's professional events.

1988	The AVP signed a three-year contract with Miller Brewing Company that provided for $4.5 million in prize money.
1990	NBC Sports televised its first AVP beach volleyball event.
1993	The AVP first trialed women's events at numerous stops on the men's tour.
1993	On September 21, the International Olympic Committee granted beach volleyball "official medal status" for the upcoming Atlanta 1996 Olympic Games.
1995	The AVP season schedule reached an all-time peak of 29 tournaments, both outdoor and indoor, held from February through September.
1996	The first Olympic Beach Volleyball competition was held at a 10,000-seat stadium in an Atlanta, Georgia park. Karch Kiraly and Kent Steffes won the gold medal with a victory over Mike Dodd and Mike Whitmarsh, the silver medalists.
1998	In a surprising move, the AVP filed for Chapter 11 bankruptcy as several sponsors left the tour, causing the prize money to be significantly reduced. The WPVA disbanded due to financial troubles.

2000	At the Sydney Olympic Games, the matches took place in beautiful Bondi Beach. The American underdogs, Dain Blanton and Eric Fonoimoana, won the gold medal.
2001	On May 31, Leonard Armato and his company Management Plus acquired the AVP. Both men's and women's competitions were combined at certain events. The new rules of rally scoring, let serve, and a reduction in court size were introduced.
2002	Karch Kiraly became the first beach volleyball player to earn more than $3 million in prize money.
2004	At the Athens Olympic Games in a 10,000-seat beach-side arena, Misty May and Kerri Walsh won the gold medal, while Holly McPeak and Elaine Youngs won the bronze.
2007	Karch Kiraly retired from the sport with a record 148 beach volleyball tournament victories. He was honored at all events during his farewell tour and received such gifts as a rocking chair, a key to the city, and a "bobble-head" statuette. Misty May-Treanor became the women's professional beach volleyball all-time wins and earnings leader, surpassing Holly McPeak.
2008	The AVP held its Hot Winter Nights indoor tour, a series of 19 events in January and February.

APPENDIX B
BEACH VOLLEYBALL TERMS

Ace
A serve that is not passable and results immediately in a point.

Angle Shot
A cross-court attack directed at an angle from one end of the offensive team's side of the net to the opposite sideline of the defensive team's court.

Chopsticks
The poking at the ball with fingertips while trying to set.

Chowder
A blatant double contact during a hand set.

Chuck
A push or throw of a ball, rather than hit or set.

Cobra
An attack using fully extended and cupped hand (like a cobra's head) to contact the ball on the top of the fingertips.

Deep Dish
A scooping up of a ball that ordinarily would have hit the ground.

Dig
The passing of a spiked or rapidly hit ball.

Dome (Facial)
A spike received to the head.

Floater
A serve that does not spin or rotate, and therefore moves in an erratic path.

Joust
A play in which two opponents make contact with the ball simultaneously above the plane of the net.

Jumbo Shrimp
A high loopy shot perfectly placed into the opposite corner.

Kill
An attack that results in an immediate point.

Kong
A one-handed block similar to the way King Kong swung at biplanes in the original movie.

Line Shot	A ball spiked down an opponent's sideline (closest to the attacker) and over or outside the block.
Nectar	A sweet play, like a near-motionless set.
Pokey	A soft attack in which the fingers are curled-up and the ball is struck with the knuckles in order to pop the ball just over the block.
Roll Shot	An attack where the ball is softly hit with a great deal of topspin so that it will clear the block and then drop quickly over it.
Shank	A poor pass that sends the ball out of play.
Sky Ball	A serve where the ball is hit underhand skywards so that as it quickly descends onto the opposite side.
Stuff (Roof)	A defensive play performed by reaching over the net and blocking the ball back at the attacker and straight to the ground.
Tool (Wipe)	A deliberate hitting of the ball off the block for a kill.
Trap	A set that is too close to the net where the attacker can easily get stuffed.
Volley Dolly	A female groupie who follows the tour.

Endnotes

Chapter 1

1. Buckheit, Mary. "Catching Up with Kerri Walsh." ESPN.com. 11 Jan. 2008 <http//espn.com>.
2. United States Olympic Committee. "Athens 2004 Video." USOC.org. Retrieved 14 Dec. 2007 <http//usoc.org>.
3. Ostler, Scott. "Scott Ostler on Kerri Walsh." The San Francisco Chronicle 13 June 2004.
4. Jay Leno Tonight Show. NBC 31 Aug. 2004.
5. Brian. "Smash Hit." Yahoo! Sports. 24 Aug. 2004 <http//sports.yahoo.com>.
6. Hartsell, Jeff. "One-on-One with Misty May-Treanor." Charleston -The Post and Courier 10 June 2007.
7. "Ten Reasons to Watch Beach Volleyball in 2007." DIG Ed.1 2007: 37.
8. Buckheit, Mary. "Easy Livin' With Misty." ESPN.com. 20 July 2007 <http//espn.com>.
9. "The Firing Line." DIG. Ed. 4 2007: 70.
10. Hamel, Larry. "A February Reach for the Beach -- Walsh, May-Treanor Boosting Volleyball with Golden Touch." Chicago Sun Times 8 February 2008 <http://suntimes.com>.

Chapter 2

1. Wegbreit, Dave. "Cuervo Celebrity Qualifier Falls Flat for Sport Insiders." Beach Volleyball Magazine 5 May 2007 <http://beachvolleyballmagazine.com>.
2. "History of Volleyball." Volleyball.com. Retrieved 10 Nov. 2007 <http://volleyball.com>
3. Buckheit, Mary. "Babes Beer and Beach Voleyball." ESPN.com 15 June 2006 <http//espn.com>
4. Hanashiro, Robert. "Icy Ad Has Sun Shining on VB Stars." USA Today 4 Mar. 2004.
5. Burke, Tom. "Cruzin'." Beach Volleyball Magazine 20 Apr. 2007.
6. An Interview with Volleyball Great Gene Selznick." Volleyball.com. Retrieved 15 Oct. 2007 <http://volleyball.com>.
7. Couvillon, Art. Sands of Times – The History of Beach Volleyball Vol #2 1970-1989. Hermosa Beach: Couvillon 2003.

8. Burke, Tom. "Cruzin'." Beach Volleyball Magazine 20 Apr 2007 <http://beachvolleyballmagazine.com>.
9. Cleary, Kevin. "Chronology of Pro Beach Volleyball and the AVP" 20 Feb. 2007.
10. Sager, Mike. "Volleyball Gods." Playboy July 1985: 122.
11. Falkoff, Robert, "Karch's Thoughts on Golden Years." AVP.com. 8 Aug. 2007 ≤http://avp.com>.

Chapter 3

1. Moore, David Leon. "U.S. Dominance Erodes on Sand." USA Today 18 Aug. 2004
2. United States Olympic Committee."Bylaws of the United States Olympic Committee."USOC.org 23 June 2006 <http://usoc.org>.
3. USAV, "About USAVolleyball." USAvolleyball.org. Retrieved 15 Sept. 2007. <http://usavolleyball.org>.
4. Ibid.
5. Ibid.
6. Soriano, Paul. "AVP Pro Beach Volleyball Tour, USA Volleyball Announce Pact." USAvolleyball.org 3 Apr. 2003. <http://usavolleyball. org>.
7. "Beach Volleyball Council to be Created." USAvolleyball.org. 10 Mar. 2005. <http://usavolleyball.org>.
8. Ibid.
9. Abrahamson, Alan. "Volleyball's Balance of Power in Question." Los Angles Times 15 Jan. 2006.
10. Miazga, Mike. "The Beach Players Vs the USA Volleyball Dispute." Volleyball Sept. 2006: 50.
11. "Beach Players/AVP File Complaint Against USA Volleyball." Volleyball Mar. 2006: 74.
12. Miazga, Mike. "The Beach Players Vs the USA Volleyball Dispute." Volleyball Sept. 2006: 50.
13. "USA Volleyball Hires Ali Wood as Director of International and High Performance Beach Programs." USAVolleyball.org. 23 Feb. 2006 <http://usavolleyball.org>.
14. "From the Service Line." Volleyball USA Fall 2007: 59.

15. "U.S. Open of Beach Volleyball Set for September 21-23 in Huntington Beach." USAvolleyball.org Retrieved 25 Sept. 2007 <http:// USAvolleyball.org>.
16. Ibid.
17. Schultz, Todd. "Change in the Air." Volleyball Sept. 2006: 20.
18. "FIVB Program Proposal - Steering Committee." FIVB.org. 20 May 2006. <http://fivb.org>.

Chapter 4

1. Sager, Mike. "Volleyball Gods." Playboy July 1985: 122.
2. Chaplin, Ralph. Lyrics from "Solidarity Forever" Jan. 1915.
3. Sager, Mike. "Volleyball Gods." Playboy July 1985: 196.
4. Cleary, Kevin. "Chronology of Pro Beach Volleyball and the AVP." 20 Feb. 2007.
5. "AVP Commish, Tour Think Big." AVP.com 14 Mar. 2007 <http:// avp.com>.
6. Cleary, Kevin. "Chronology of Pro Beach Volleyball and the AVP" 20 Feb. 2007.
7. Ibid.
8. Couvillon, Art. Sands of Times – The History of Beach Volleyball Vol #3. Hermosa Beach: Couvillon 2004: 59.
9. According to several sources, his resignation was due his family deciding to move away from California because of an earthquake that destroyed his home.
10. Lefton, Terry. "Sand in Their Face – The Game Quarterly," Brandweek 20 Apr. 1998.
11. Ibid.
12. Ibid.
13. Ibid.
14. Ibid.
15. AVP. "AVP Suspends Steffes." AVP Press Release. 27 Nov. 1998.
16. Lefton, Terry. "Honda, Miller Spike AVP As League Mulls Fate." Brandweek 5 Oct. 1998.
17. Ibid.
18. AVP, Inc. AVP Press Release 3 Feb. 1999.
19. Bresnahan, Mike. "New AVP Tackles Some Old Problems." Los Angeles Times 23 May 2002.

20. Bresnahan, Mike. "Gold Medal Winners Leaving the AVP Tour Acrimoniously." Los Angeles Times 6 Apr. 2001.
21. Lefton, Terry. "Sand in Their Face – The Game Quarterly." Brandweek 20 Apr. 1998.

Chapter 5

1. Crossman, Nate. "AVP Is Alive and Well After Brush with Extinction." The Patriot Ledger 16 Aug. 2007.
2. Bresnahan, Mike. "Volleyball Deal May Spike Interest." Los Angeles Times 8 Apr. 2001.
3. Crenshaw, Solomon. "Flexing its Muscles, Bigger Prize Purses, Growing Fan Base Illustrate Beach Volleyball's Rise in Popularity." Birmingham News 14 July 2006.
4. In 2001, the court was reduced from an 18 m. x 9 m. size to a 16m x 8 m size for use in AVP tournaments.
5. Bresnahan, Mike. "Volleyball Deal May Spike Interest." Los Angeles Times 8 Apr. 2001.
6. Smith, Marcia C. "Armato Taking It to the Beach." Ocean County Register 28 May 2002.
7. "Q & A – Leonard Armato" Volleyball Aug. 2004: 35.
8. Anderson, Kelli. "A New Beachhead." Sports Illustrated 3 Sept. 2001.
9. Smith, Marcia C. "Armato Taking It to the Beach." Ocean County Register 28 May 2002.
10. Satzman, Darrell. "Ex-Agent Armato Bounces Back to Beach Volleyball." Los Angeles Business Journal 16 June 2003.
11. "Q & A – Leonard Armato" Volleyball Aug. 2004: 35.
12. AVP, Inc. AVP Press Release April 2005.
13. Crossman, Nate. "AVP Is Alive and Well After Brush with Extinction." The Patriot Ledger 16 Aug. 2007.
14. AVP, Inc. "10KSB SEC Filing." SEC.gov, 17 April 2006, <http://sec.gov>.
15. AVP, Inc. AVP Press Release 4 Apr 2007.
16. Diker Management, LLC. Letter to AVP Board of Directors 10 Apr 2007.
17. Amtrust Capital Management. Letter to AVP Board of Directors 1 July 2007.

18. Miazga, Mike. "Proposed AVP Merger Drawing Shareholder Ire." Volleyball July 2007: 18.
19. AVP, Inc. "AVP and Shamrock Terminate Merger Agreement." SEC 8K Filing 5 Sept. 2007.
20. Scarr, Mike. "Hot Winter Nights Set to Start." AVP.com. 8 Jan. 2008 <http://avp.com>.

Chapter 6

1. "The Firing Line." DIG. Ed. 4 2007: 70.
2. Mason, Nancy. "Nancy Mason on Partner Swapping." AVP.com. 25 May 2005. <http://AVP.com>.
3. Bikinis are required by the AVP – unless the weather is cold, windy, or rainy. In which case, women have worn leggings and long sleeve tees to compete in. Examples: Lake Tahoe, NV in 2006 and Boston, MA in 2007.
4. Ryan, John. "The Gold Standard - Walsh Helps Local Youths." San Jose Mercury News 5 June 2005.
5. Buckheit, Mary. "Catching Up with Kerri Walsh." ESPN.com. 1 Jan. 2008. <http//espn.com>.
6. Kane Colleen. "California Gleamin'." The Cincinnati Enquirer 2 July 2005.
7. Casey, Tim. "AVP Continues Growing." Sacramento Bee 19 June 2006.
8. Karbo, Karen and Gabby Reece. Big Girl in the Middle Crown Publishers, 1997.
9. Price, Shawn. "Tough Question for Women of AVP." Ocean County Register 22 Aug. 2005.
10. Ibid.

Chapter 7

1. Dyer, Mike. "AVP Wants to Emulate the Success of NASCAR." Cincinnati Enquirer 2 July 2005.
2. "2007 AVP Pro Beach Volleyball Overview" Mikemorrison.us Retrieved 3 Mar. 2008, <http://mikemorrison.us>.
3. Anderson, Kelli. "A New Beachhead." Sports Illustrated 3 Sept. 2001.

4. Mulhern, Mike. "ESPN Shrugs Off Dwindling NASCAR Ratings." Scripps News 22 Nov. 2007.

5. Hoffer, Richard. "Dig This." Sports Illustrated 19 Aug. 2002: 46.

6. Bissell, Kimberly and Duke, Andrea M. "Angles of Women's Beach Volleyball During the 2004 Summer Olympics." Journal of Promotion Management Volume 13, Numbers 1-2, 28 November 2007: 35-53.

7. AVP, Inc. "10KSB SEC Filing." SEC.gov, 17 April 2006, <http://sec.gov>.

8. Bresnahan, Mike. "'New' AVP Tackles Some Old Problems." Los Angeles Times 23 May 2002.

9. AVP, Inc. "AVP Announces First Live Broadcast of Tour Events on Fox." AVP Press Release 21 Feb 2006.

10. "AVP hires CAA Sports for Cable Deal and More." Sports Business Journal 12 Dec. 2007.

Chapter 8

1. Lefton, Terry. "Sand in Their Face – The Game Quarterly." Brandweek 20 Apr. 1998.

2. Ibid.

3. MacMillan, Carrie "Digging for Sponsors," Promo Magazine.com. 2 June 2003 <http://promomagazine.com>.

4. Ibid.

5. "Q&A: Marketing AVP Volleyball Is Nothing But Net (Gains)." Brandweek 3 Apr. 2005.

6. Kane Colleen. "California Gleamin'." The Cincinnati Enquirer 2 July 2005.

7. AVP, Inc. "AVP Pro Beach Volleyball Completes Successful 2005 Season With 48% Increase in Fan Base - Scarborough Sports Marketing Confirms That AVP Tour is Fastest Growing Sports Property." AVP Press Release 4 Nov. 2005.

8. Smith, Marcia. "Beach Volleyball Back in Business." Ocean County Register 30 May 2006.

9. Miazga, Mike. "Q&A – Leonard Armato." Volleyball May 2004: 31.

10. MacMillan, Carrie. "Digging for Sponsors." Promo Magazine.com. 2 June 2003 <http://promomagazine.com>.

11. AVP, Inc. "Cuervo Returns as Official Sponsor of AVP Pro Beach Volleyball Tour." AVP Press Release 9 Jan. 2006.

12. AVP. "AVP's Sports Sponsorship Symposium." <u>AVP Press Release</u> 27 Sept. 2006.

13. Ibid.

Chapter 9

1. Stolfus, Hans. "The Groveler's Report," <u>DIG</u> Ed. 6 2006: 27.

2. AVP, Inc. "10KSB SEC Filing." SEC.gov, 17 Apr. 2006, <http://sec. gov>.

3. United States. U.S. Census Bureau. "U.S. Census Bureau Poverty Thresholds 2007." <u>Census.gov</u> 2007 <http://census.gov/hhes/www/ poverty/threshld/thresh07.html>.

4. Miazga, Mike. "American Nomad." <u>Volleyball</u> Jan. 2007: 22.

5. Akers, Angie. "Deal With It," <u>Volleyball</u> June 2007: 62.

6. Stolfus, Hans. "Finding a Voice. " <u>Volleyball.com</u>. 18 Jan. 2008 <http://volleyball.com>.

7. MacMillan, Carrie. "Digging for Sponsors." <u>Promo Magazine.com</u>. 2 June 2003 <http://promomagazine.com>.

8. Villa, Walter. "Gibb Eyes More Than a Title." <u>AVP.com</u>. 13 Apr. 2007 <http://avp.com>.

9. Fuerbringer, Matt. "Fuerby Muses on Training." <u>AVP.com</u>. 25 May 2005 <http://avp.com>.

10. AVP, Inc. "AVP 2007 Crocs Tour Launch Party." <u>AVP Press Release</u> 29 Mar. 2007

11. "Armato Interview." DIG Ed. 6 2006: 34.

12. Ibid.

13. Ibid.

14. Villa, Walter. "Zartman's Born for the Beach." <u>AVP.com</u>. 5 Dec. 2007 <http://avp.com>.

15. Iovineo, Stephanie. "Misty May-Treanor: Solid Gold," <u>Womensportsfoundation.org</u> Sept. 2007 <http:// womensportsfoundation.org>.

16. Kinmartin, Patrick. "For Lindquist, Life is at the Beach." <u>The Daily Trojan</u> 28 Apr 2005.

17. "The Way it Was." <u>Beach Volleyball Magazine</u> Oct. 2006: 61.

18. Sleeper, John. "Volleyball Tour in Everett: Far from Home, Players Become Friends, Competitors." <u>Herald Columnist</u> 15 Feb. 2008.

19. Murray, Colleen. "Goals for 2007." <u>AVP.com</u>. 2 Jan. 2007 <http://avp.com>.

20. AVP, Inc. "DIG Show - Tampa Tournament." <u>AVP.com</u>. May 2007 <http://avp.com>.

21. Stolfus, Hans. "The Groveler's Report." <u>DIG</u> Ed. 6 2006.

Chapter 10

1. Schmetzer, Mark. "Top Seeds Remain Unstoppable." <u>The Cincinnati Enquirer</u> 3 Sept. 2007.

2. Kiefaber, Adam. "Favorites Make Mason Sand Their Playground." <u>The Cincinnati Post</u> 3 Sept. 2007.

3. Zant, John. "To have and to hold: Finding the Right Partner." <u>Santa Barbara News-Press</u> 5 May 2005.

4. Zuvela, Matt. "Q&A With Blanton." <u>AVP.com</u>. 30 Jan. 2007 <http://avp.com>.

5. "AVP Interview." <u>The Early Show</u> CBS. 17 Aug. 2006.

6. Berg, Aimee. "Little Room for Shorter Players on the Beach." <u>AVP.com</u>. 25 Aug. 2007 <http://avp.com>.

7. "Beach Digs – A Few Days at the Beach." <u>Volleyball USA</u> Summer 2004: 7.

8. Zant, John. "To have and to hold: Finding the Right Partner." <u>Santa Barbara News-Press</u> 5 May 2005.

9. Boyko, Lara. "Longevity." <u>Volleyball</u> May 2004: 24.

10. Villa. Walter. "Sister Act: The Lindquists." <u>AVP.com</u>. 11 Apr. 2007. <http://avp.com>.

11. Cantrell, Blake. "Interview with Johnny Jamba." <u>DIG</u> Ed. 5 2007: 60.

12. Katzowitz, Josh. "Golden Girls 50 Game Streak Ends." <u>The Cincinnati Post</u> 2 July 2005.

13. Miazga, Mike. "Breakthrough," <u>Volleyball</u> Nov. 2005: 41.

14. Boyko, Lara. "AVP Veteran Nancy Mason is Beginning Her 13th Professional Season and is Enjoying the Ride." <u>Volleyball</u> May 2006: 39.

15. Swan, Darren. "Jennings, Fuerbringer Reunite." <u>AVP.com</u>. 3 Aug. 2007. <http://avp.com>.

16. Ibid.

17. "Men's Side to Feature New Look." <u>Volleyball</u> March 2005: 27.

18. Murray, Steve. "Old Friends Column." <u>Midweek.com</u>. 19 Oct. 2005 <http://midweek.com>.
19. Akers, Angie. "Deal With It." <u>Volleyball</u>. June 2007: 62.
20. Sanders, Bill. "Three Things on Boss' Mind: Weather, Wacholder and Walsh Are All Concerns." <u>AVP.com</u>. 8 June 2007 <http://avp.com>.
21. Berg, Aimee. "Little Room for Short Players on the Beach." <u>The New York Times</u> 25 Aug. 2007.
22. "One-On-One – Jeff and Dianne." <u>DIG</u> Ed. 4 2007: 60.
23. Moya, Monique. "Boss Ross Mix It Up in Vegas." <u>AVP.com</u>. 7 Sept. 2007. <http://avp.com>.
24. Sims, Kelly. "The Little Player with the Big Game." <u>DIG</u> Ed. 4 2007: 32.
25. Mason, Nancy. "Nancy Mason on Partner Swapping." <u>AVP.com</u>. 5 May 2005 <http://avp.com>.
26. "Volleyball Icon Holly McPeak Reflects on Winning the Bronze." <u>USAVolleyball.org</u>. Retrieved 10 Sept. 2007 <http://usavolleyball.org>.
27. Villa, Walter. "McPeak to Hang 'em Up After 2008." <u>AVP.com</u>. 7 Apr. 2007 <http://avp.com>.
28. Scarr, Mike. "AVP Media Day Kicks Off '07 Season." <u>AVP.com</u>. 29 Mar. 2007 <http://avp.com>.
29. "Hitting Stride." <u>DIG</u> Ed. 4 2007: 47.

Chapter 11

1. Smith, Marcia. "Wacholder Digs Beach Game Again." <u>Ocean City Register</u> 9 Aug. 2005.
2. "Five Tips with Albert Hannemann." <u>AVP.com</u>. 12 Jan. 2007 <http://avp.com>.
3. Boyko, Lara. "Sticking Together." <u>Volleyball</u> Aug. 2006: 44.
4. Murray, Colleen. "Ross' Beach Efforts Pay Off." AVP.com. 22 Apr. 2007 <http://avp.com>.
5. Moyal Monique. "AVP Welcomes New Breed of Players." <u>AVP.com</u>. 19 Mar. 2007 <http://avp.com>.

6. Nygaard, Jeff. "Five Tips With Jeff Nygaard." AVP.com. 15 Dec. 2006 <http://avp.com>.

7. "One-On-One – Jeff and Dianne," DIG Ed. 4 2007: 60.

8. Strauss, Doug. "Volleyball is a Year Round Business." AVP.com. 11 Mar. 2005 <http://avp.com>.

9. Nygaard, Jeff. "Jeff Nygaard on the 2005 AVP Season." AVP.com. 7 Apr. 2005 <http://avp.com>.

10. Jennings, Casey. "Casey Jennings Testimonial." Budokon.com. Retrieved 10 Aug. 2007 <http://budokon.com>.

11. Falkoff, Robert. "Rogers a Mental Giant." AVP.com. 2 Apr. 2007 <http://avp.com>.

12. Villa, Walter. "Logan Tom Enjoys a Breakthrough." AVP.com. 29 May 2007. <http://avp.com>

13. Hastings, Jon. "A New Challenge." DIG Ed. 3 2007: 4.

14. Hoffarth, Tom. "Sun Has a Dark Side for AVP Pros." Los Angeles Daily News 21 May 2007.

15. Patterson, Don. "Too Tough." DIG Ed. 1 2004: 33.

16. Scarr, Mike. "Dodd Enjoying Second AVP Career." AVP.com. 15 Sept. 2007 <http://avp.com>.

Chapter 12

1. Smith, Marcia. "Beach Volleyball Back in Business." Ocean County Register 30 May 2006.

2. Wong, Scott and Katie Nelson. "Pro Beach Volleyball Shifting Play from Tempe to Glendale." The Arizona Republic 4 Jan. 2007.

3. "Beach Boss." DIG Ed.6 2006: 34.

4. AVP. "10KSB SEC Filing." SEC.gov. 17 Apr. 2006 <http://sec.gov>.

5. Scarr, Mike. "Building a Beach at a Ballpark." AVP.com. 19 Apr. 2007 <http://avp.com>.

6. Bowman, Phillip. "Olson, Ring Battling from Loss." AVP.com. 17 June 2007 <http://avp.com>.

7. Raimondi, Marc. "Weather Affects Last Two Tour Stops." AVP.com. 25 Aug. 2007 <http://avp.com>.

8. Zuvela, Matt. "Not All Beaches Are Created Equal." AVP.com. 1 Jan. 2007. <http://avp.com>.

9. "Tropical Storm Plays Havoc in Tampa." <u>AVP.com</u>. 2 Jun.2007 <http://avp.com>.

Chapter 13

1. Scarr, Mike. "First Things First for Men in Qualifier." <u>AVP.com</u>. 9 Aug. 2007 <http://avp.com.>.
2. Falkoff, Robert. "Tramblie Battles Injury, Moves On." <u>AVP.com</u>. 19 Apr. 2007 <http://avp.com>.
3. Falkoff, Robert. "Novacek Falls Early in Qualifier." <u>AVP.com</u>. 19 Apr. 2007 <http://avp.com>.
4. Katzowitz, Josh. "Golden Girls 50 Game Streak Ends." <u>The Cincinnati Post</u> 2 July 2005.
5. "Intimidation." <u>AVP.com</u>. 2 Feb. 2007 <http://avp.com>.
6. Falkoff, Robert. "Shocking Exit of Metzger, Lambert." <u>AVP.com</u>. 20 Apr. 2007 <http://avp.com>.
7. Ibid.
8. Vargas, Nicole. "Top Men's Seed Tested; Women's No. 1 Coasts." <u>San Diego Union Tribune</u> 12 June 2005.
9. Miller, Jay N. "It's a Rough Road for the Losers." <u>The Patriot Ledger</u> 18 Aug. 2007.
10. Mason, Nancy. "Nancy Mason is Talking AVP Officiating." <u>AVP.com</u>. 9 May 2005. <http://avp.com>.
11. Boyko, Lara. "Third Time Can Be Charm or Curse." <u>AVP.com</u>. 15 Sept. 2007 <http://avp.com>.
12. Nygaard, Jeff. "Player's Corner with Jeff Nygaard." <u>AVP.com</u>. 17 Aug. 2005 <http://avp.com>.
13. Falkoff, Robert. "Ivy-Lowe, New Force on Women's Tour." <u>AVP.com</u>. 8 June 2007 <http://avp.com>.
14. Emerson Lake & Palmer. Lyrics from "Karn Evil 9 - 1st Impression, Part 2". Manticore Records.
15. Kaufman, Amy. "Worming His Way to the Top." <u>AVP.com</u>. 4 Apr. 2006 <http://avp.com>.
16. Miller, Jay. "Dalhausser, Rogers Hold Off Threat." <u>The Patriot Ledger</u> 18 Aug. 2007.

17. Schmetzer, Mark. "Top Seeds Remain Unstoppable." The Cincinnati Enquirer 3 Sept. 2007.
18. Crossman, Nate. "AVP is Alive and Well After Brush with Extinction." The Patriot Ledger 16 Aug. 2007.

Chapter 14

1. Mahoney, Brian. "Smash Hit." Yahoo! Sports. 24 Aug. 2004 <http// sports.yahoo.com>.
2. Wilson, Bernie. "Shaq's Agent Revives Pro Beach Volleyball Tour." CBC Sports. 9 June 2001 <http//cbc.ca>.
3. AVP. "AVP, Inc. Announces 2007 Third Quarter Financial Results." AVP Press Release 12 Nov. 2007.
4. Hamel, Larry. "A February Reach for the Beach -- Walsh, May-Treanor Boosting Volleyball with Golden Touch." Chicago Sun Times 8 Feb. 2008.

Acknowledgments

During this journey, several people were instrumental along the way.

My heartfelt gratitude goes out to Bijan Bayne and Hildie Block for their support in the initial, conceptual stage, Kevin Quirk for his ongoing guidance and critique, Peter Bowerman and Daniel Stevens for their publishing advice, Ryan Gray for offering freelance beach volleyball opportunities, and *JustYourType.biz* for the book design. All made this dream come true.

Special thanks to Dennis Wagner, the creator of the *Beach Volleyball Database* that I continually relied on for researching and fact-finding, Art Couvillon for providing pictures and publishing of the "Sands of Time" series of books that detailed the history of beach volleyball, and Kevin Cleary, the founding President of the AVP, for chronicling the AVP history in a convenient outline.

I greatly appreciate all the AVP players and staff members who met with me at tournaments, in hotel lobbies, and over the phone on endless occasions to discuss the professional beach volleyball scene.

Love and special thanks to my wife, Jeanne, whose ongoing patience and assistance were invaluable; to my daughter, Emily, whose research and promotional assistance were very helpful; and to the rest my family for all their support over the years, Walter, Martha, Jim, Mark, and Brent.

Index